# RETHINKING HEALTH SECRETS

Exposing the Real Causes of
Modern Illness and the Protocols
to Reset Your Health Naturally

Moonlit Feather Books

*Modern illness isn't just personal: it's systemic*

# Table of Contents

# Part I — The Hidden Crisis

You did what you were told. You sought help, followed the advice, made the changes they recommended. You tried the foods, the supplements, the routines. But your health didn't respond the way you hoped. The truth? It's not your fault. The system was built to manage symptoms, not to ask why they began in the first place.

Part I is about what no one warned you: that the system you turned to for help was never designed to get you well. It was designed to keep you managed, just enough to function, not enough to thrive.

In this section, we shine a light on the silent incentives, the economic machinery, and the deeply ingrained beliefs that keep millions trapped in cycles of fatigue, inflammation, misdiagnosis, and dismissal. We expose the gap between real healing and what passes for "healthcare" today. You'll see how convenience became more profitable than purity, how chronic illness became a business model, and how symptoms became normalized—until you stopped questioning them.

This is not about blame. It's about clarity.

Before you can rebuild trust in your body, you must first understand why that trust was eroded in the first place.

# Chapter 1: Trapped in a Sickcare Economy

## How the System Profits from Sickness

When we think of health care, most of us picture something noble: doctors helping patients, hospitals saving lives, breakthrough medications curing illness. And while there's truth to those images, the full picture is far more complicated. Beneath the surface of what appears to be a system dedicated to healing lies a deeply embedded infrastructure of profit, one that often thrives more on the existence of chronic illness than on its resolution.

At the center of this is the simple truth: **there is more money in managing illness than in curing it**. Chronic conditions like diabetes, autoimmune disorders, heart disease, and fatigue-related syndromes generate billions in recurring revenue every year through pharmaceuticals, medical devices, tests, and specialist visits. If someone gets cured, the income stream ends. But if their symptoms are merely controlled—just enough to stay afloat—they stay within the system indefinitely.

This isn't a conspiracy; it's a structural reality. From insurance companies to pharmaceutical giants, the incentives are stacked around prolonged treatment, not root-cause resolution. A single surgery may cost tens of thousands once, but a person on medication for the rest of their life could generate hundreds of thousands in profit over decades. Multiply that by millions of patients and it becomes clear: chronic disease is a lucrative business model.

Marketing plays a powerful role in keeping this engine running. Many people don't realize that pharmaceutical companies spend more on advertising and "doctor outreach" than on research and development. That means more money goes into shaping perception—both patient and physician—than into solving the deeper causes of disease. Direct-to-consumer ads (which are legal only in the U.S. and New Zealand) push patients to "ask their doctor" about the latest drugs. And doctors, often overwhelmed by packed schedules and limited appointment time, lean heavily on pharmaceutical reps and pre-approved treatment protocols.

But what if the real solution isn't a pill? What if the underlying cause of brain fog, joint pain, low energy, or inflammation lies in nutrition, toxic exposure, stress overload, or gut dysfunction? These questions rarely reach center stage because the answers aren't profitable in the same way. No one is raking in billions by telling you to get clean sleep, reduce processed food, or manage hidden mold exposure. In fact, if widespread root-cause healing took place, many sectors of the health economy would shrink dramatically.

It's important to be precise here: the system isn't evil. But **it is misaligned**. Most individual doctors and nurses genuinely care. Many scientists dedicate their lives to improving health. But they're working inside a machine that rewards volume over depth, speed over accuracy, and treatment over transformation. It's a system that financially incentivizes short-term fixes and repeat prescriptions, not long-term restoration.

And this model extends beyond medicine. Think of processed food companies that engineer products to be hyper-palatable, even addictive, while simultaneously funding wellness campaigns. Or chemical manufacturers whose products end up in your body through plastics, packaging, or pollution—and who sponsor studies to downplay the risks. Or even gyms and wellness apps that capitalize on guilt, offering surface solutions instead of helping people rebuild foundational health.

This isn't just about corporate greed. It's about a widespread **cultural conditioning**—one where quick fixes are normalized and slow healing is inconvenient. We're trained to think that if there's no instant answer, the problem must be "in our head." Or worse, unsolvable.

But what if the truth is more complex—and more empowering?

And that complexity is exactly where the system falls short. Because chronic conditions don't fit neatly into a pill-per-day solution. Fatigue, brain fog, and inflammation often arise from an intersection of subtle factors: food intolerances, chronic stress, gut imbalances, environmental toxins, sleep disruption, and emotional suppression. These are not exotic or rare problems—they're everyday realities. But they're not part of the dominant treatment model because they don't generate recurring billing codes or billion-dollar patents.

What's more troubling is how this misalignment shapes medical education. Most medical schools in the U.S. offer **less than 25 hours of nutrition training across the entire curriculum**. And yet, conditions like Type 2 diabetes, heart disease, and even cognitive decline are intimately linked to what we eat. Many health professionals are simply never taught to consider the root cause beyond the most obvious, testable metrics. They learn to look for what can be diagnosed and coded quickly—because that's how the system measures "efficiency."

Insurance plays a pivotal role here. Reimbursements are structured around brief visits, tests, and drug regimens. Deep-diving into a patient's toxic load, stress levels, sleep quality, or trauma history takes time. Time that isn't billable. So instead of tracking what truly changes outcomes, the system tracks what's measurable and monetizable.

This doesn't just affect what patients are prescribed—it also affects what they believe about their bodies. When someone feels dismissed or rushed through the process, they internalize the idea that **their symptoms aren't real** or that **nothing can be done**. Over time, they stop asking questions. They settle. They accept feeling half-alive as the norm.

And then there's the influence of industry-funded research. While there are many brilliant and ethical scientists in the field, it's an open secret that **most major studies are funded or influenced by the same companies that stand to profit from their outcomes**. That's not inherently corrupt, but it does raise a critical issue: when funding shapes research design, data interpretation, and public messaging, the line between science and marketing begins to blur.

Take for example how cholesterol was demonized for decades while sugar quietly escaped scrutiny. Or how the conversation around inflammation was largely silenced until it became undeniable. Or how pesticides, plastics, and environmental estrogens are still underplayed in mainstream conversations despite growing evidence of their biological impact. These are not minor oversights. They reflect how **selective visibility** shapes public understanding of health.

The system profits not just by selling solutions, but by limiting the menu of acceptable problems. If your symptoms can't be explained within the framework of lab results and ICD-10 codes, the default explanation becomes psychosomatic. You're anxious. You're stressed. You're "just getting older." And so, the loop continues: suppressed symptoms, partial treatments, new side effects, more appointments, new prescriptions.

What's often missing is the encouragement to truly investigate. To ask: *What is my body trying to tell me? What patterns have I normalized? What inputs am I not even aware of?* Most people don't even know where to begin—not because they're lazy or unmotivated, but because the system hasn't empowered them to understand their health outside of institutional terms.

But the reality is, once people begin to see the patterns—how inflammation is linked to gut health, how brain fog connects to food chemicals, how fatigue relates to stress hormones and environmental exposures—they can start to reclaim a sense of agency. Not magical cures. Not overnight transformations. But clear, actionable insights that were never part of the conversation.

Understanding how the system profits from sickness isn't about blaming every practitioner or distrusting every treatment. It's about recognizing that a machine designed for crisis management and revenue generation is not built for holistic healing. It never was.

And until we acknowledge that, we'll keep askin

# The Symptoms You've Been Taught to Ignore

We live in a world where discomfort has become background noise—where fatigue is shrugged off, brain fog is "just a rough day," and digestive issues are normalized with memes and jokes. Most people have come to accept a baseline level of dysfunction as "just life." But what if these symptoms aren't just annoying interruptions? What if they're your body's most intelligent form of communication—signals that something deeper needs attention?

From a young age, we're taught to override symptoms. Got a headache? Take a painkiller. Feeling anxious? Distract yourself. Bloated? Must be something you ate—don't think too much about it. The underlying message is subtle but consistent: symptoms are a nuisance, not a clue. This conditioning runs deep, and it's reinforced by cultural habits, marketing, and even well-meaning doctors who often lack the time or framework to explore root causes.

But symptoms aren't random. They're information. They're your body's internal diagnostics. And the reason they've been so easy to ignore—or suppress—is because we haven't been trained to interpret them. We've been taught to label them instead. And once something has a label, we tend to stop being curious.

Take chronic fatigue, for example. It's so common that many people don't even bring it up anymore. They assume it's because they're not sleeping well, working too hard, getting older. Maybe they've even had blood tests come back "normal." So they push through it. But persistent fatigue isn't just about low energy—it's often a signal of underlying inflammation, mitochondrial dysfunction, hormone imbalances, or nutritional depletion. Ignoring it may not be dangerous immediately, but over time, it robs you of clarity, mood stability, and resilience.

Or consider brain fog—that hazy, disconnected feeling that makes it hard to focus or recall words. It's not a diagnosable condition in most settings, yet it's one of the most common early warning signs of systemic stress. Brain fog can point to blood sugar instability, sleep disturbances, gut-brain axis disruption, or even subtle neuroinflammation. Left unaddressed, it can lead to decreased productivity, increased anxiety, and even early cognitive decline.

Another widely ignored symptom is bloating. Not the occasional after-meal fullness, but persistent bloating that becomes part of your daily life. It's often chalked up to "bad digestion" or "eating too fast," but chronic bloating can reveal deep imbalances in your gut flora, food sensitivities, or impaired enzyme production. And since the gut is at the core of immune regulation, emotional processing, and hormonal function, ignoring this signal can trigger a ripple effect across nearly every system in the body.

Skin issues like adult acne, eczema, or mysterious rashes are also frequently minimized. They're treated with creams or makeup, and rarely seen for what they often are: reflections of internal stress, toxic burden, or immune dysregulation. The skin is not a separate entity—it's an extension of the gut and liver. When those systems are overburdened, the skin steps in to offload waste. That breakout or flare-up? It's not just cosmetic. It's a message.

But we've been taught to disconnect from these messages. And the consequences aren't just physical—they're emotional too. When someone constantly feels "off" but has been told everything is "fine," they begin to question their instincts. They start to believe that maybe it's all in their head. That maybe they're overreacting. That maybe they should just learn to live with it.

This learned dismissal becomes a barrier to healing. Because to heal, you have to believe that your symptoms matter. That they're not overreactions, but intelligent signals. And that you're not broken—you're just out of alignment with what your body actually needs.

When someone begins to truly listen to their symptoms, an entirely new language of the body starts to unfold—one built not on fear, but on curiosity. They stop asking "How do I get rid of this?" and start asking "Why is this happening?" That shift opens the door to deeper insight, more aligned choices, and long-term resolution instead of short-term relief.

A woman who's been dealing with hormonal acne for years might finally stop blaming her skin and start investigating what her cycle, stress levels, and liver function are trying to say. She might realize that it's not just about what she puts *on* her face—but what her body is trying to excrete *through* it. And once she sees the connection, everything changes. She doesn't just treat the surface anymore. She supports the system beneath it.

Or a man who has accepted daily acid reflux as normal finally pauses to ask what his digestion is protesting. Is it the pace of his meals? A loss of stomach acid, not an excess? Chronic stress stealing energy from his gut? He realizes that the body isn't making a mistake—it's raising a red flag. And instead of reaching automatically for the antacid, he begins to slow down, chew more, remove irritants, support digestion. Relief doesn't come from suppression, but from participation.

This kind of healing isn't instant, and it isn't flashy. It doesn't look like a miracle pill or a dramatic before-and-after. It looks like someone re-entering a relationship with their own biology—gradually, attentively, and with a sense of responsibility. They stop outsourcing every decision and begin collecting data from their own lived experience. They track how they feel after certain meals, how their energy responds to stress, how their sleep shifts when they stay off screens at night. And slowly, the picture becomes clearer.

Even more profound than the physical benefits is the psychological shift. People who begin to trust their symptoms regain a sense of sovereignty that the health system often unintentionally strips away. They stop feeling like helpless patients in a broken system and start becoming partners in their own recovery. And that mindset shift alone can spark transformation. Because when someone believes their body is wise—not defective—they begin to treat it with respect, not resentment.

This isn't about rejecting modern medicine. It's about expanding the definition of what health truly means. It's about bringing awareness to the spaces that conventional care sometimes overlooks—not out of neglect, but because of time constraints, systemic pressures, or outdated models. It's also about noticing that symptoms often surface long before anything shows up in lab results. Waiting for a diagnosis before acting means missing the early signals. And in many cases, those signals are the only warning the body will give before more serious breakdowns occur. That's why learning to decode these subtle messages is so powerful. The earlier we recognize them, the earlier we can intervene. Not with panic, but with precision. Not with fear, but with a sense of collaboration. That ache, that drop in energy, that recurring rash—it's your biology tapping you on the shoulder, trying to get your attention.

Some of the most common symptoms people have been taught to ignore are also the ones that hold the most insight: difficulty waking up in the morning, crashing in the afternoon, needing caffeine just to function, feeling puffy or swollen without explanation, recurring headaches, irritability after eating, restless sleep, irregular cycles, low libido. None of these exist in a vacuum. They're not personal flaws or random annoyances. They're interconnected and systemic.

And the truth is, many people don't need more discipline or stronger willpower—they need better understanding. Once that understanding is in place, the motivation to support the body flows naturally. There's no need for perfection, just consistent attention. And in that space of attention, healing often begins.

Learning to honor symptoms as messengers doesn't mean obsessing over every sensation. It means staying aware, staying curious, and staying responsive. It means asking better questions, even when the answers aren't immediately available. And it means remembering that your body is always speaking—even when the world around you is trying to mute the sound.

Once that awareness is awake, it doesn't go back to sleep. It becomes a lifelong compass. One that doesn't just help you manage your health—but helps you reclaim it.

# Why You're Still Tired, Foggy, and Inflamed

You wake up tired, push through the day in a mental fog, and feel like your body is subtly inflamed from the inside out. You've tried the basics—more sleep, less sugar, even supplements—but nothing seems to move the needle. The frustrating part is that your bloodwork might be "normal." Your doctor may even tell you that you're fine. But you're not. Something inside you knows that your body is trying to speak—and it's time to listen.

Fatigue, brain fog, and inflammation aren't random. They're signals. And when they persist, it means something deeper is at play. The problem is that most systems only address the symptoms, not the underlying cause. You get recommendations like "just exercise more," "manage your stress," or "cut carbs"—which might help a little but don't resolve the root issue. And you're left spinning, wondering if this is just the way life is now.

But this isn't about you being lazy, weak, or imagining things. It's about hidden burdens the modern body carries every day. Fatigue isn't a character flaw. Brain fog isn't a moral failing. Chronic inflammation isn't bad luck. They're the consequence of a system that's overworked, undernourished, and constantly bombarded—by food, environment, and even information.

Start with energy. Real, sustainable energy doesn't come from caffeine or sugar spikes. It comes from efficient mitochondria—those tiny engines in your cells that convert food and oxygen into fuel. But today, those engines are often damaged or overloaded. Why? Poor-quality food. Toxins. Chronic stress. Lack of restorative sleep. Even low-grade infections or hidden inflammation can impair your cells' ability to make energy. So when you feel drained, it's not just a lack of motivation. It's biology. And it's reversible—once you understand the layers beneath it. Brain fog is similar. That hazy, slow, disconnected feeling isn't just mental. It's often a reflection of physical issues—blood sugar dysregulation, inflammation in the gut-brain axis, or nutrient deficiencies. Most people don't know that the brain is incredibly sensitive to what happens in the body. A leaky gut, even without digestive symptoms, can trigger immune responses that affect cognition. Swings in blood sugar can make you feel like you're crashing mid-sentence. And chronic exposure to ultra-processed food can slowly dull your clarity—not because you're getting older, but because your brain is inflamed.

And then there's the inflammation itself. It doesn't always show up as pain. Sometimes it's subtle: puffiness, mood swings, poor recovery, skin issues, low-grade anxiety, or just a sense of heaviness. Inflammation is your immune system's way of signaling distress. It's trying to clean up, to defend. But when the threats are constant—processed food, synthetic chemicals, disrupted sleep, unresolved trauma—your body never gets the chance to return to baseline. The result? You feel like you're always "off," even if you can't pinpoint why.

And the worst part? This is now considered normal. We've normalized dysfunction. You're told that it's just aging. That everyone feels like this. That you should be grateful your labs are normal. But health isn't defined by what's *not* wrong—it's defined by how alive and aligned you feel.

The accumulation of stressors in the body isn't always obvious. It's not about a single dramatic event. It's the slow build-up: the chemicals in your shampoo, the late-night screen time, the processed snacks, the skipped meals, the chronic low-grade worry you barely notice anymore. One by one, these micro-stressors pile up—and eventually, they tip the scale. Your system goes from resilient to reactive. From adaptive to overloaded.

And once that tipping point is reached, it becomes incredibly difficult to feel rested, clear, or stable. Not because your body is broken, but because it's constantly trying to survive in conditions it wasn't designed for. Imagine trying to run complex software on an overheated computer with too many tabs open—it slows, lags, maybe crashes. That's your biology on modern life.

One of the key systems under pressure is the **hypothalamic-pituitary-adrenal (HPA) axis**—your body's main stress response network. When it's activated too often, your cortisol rhythms get disrupted. You might wake up feeling groggy but wired at night. Or feel flat and unmotivated all day. Over time, this dysregulation doesn't just affect your mood—it impacts your blood sugar, digestion, hormones, and immune response. Chronic fatigue is often tied not to lack of energy production, but to misfired stress signals that are draining your reserves behind the scenes. Another overlooked factor is **low-grade inflammation in the gut and brain**. The gut lining is meant to be semi-permeable, allowing nutrients through and keeping toxins out. But when it's constantly exposed to food additives, stress hormones, or antibiotics, it begins to leak—literally. This allows unwanted substances into the bloodstream, triggering immune reactions and inflammation. What many people think of as "mental" fatigue or fog is actually rooted in these immune responses. It's not all in your head. It's in your gut. And your brain is responding accordingly.

Then there's **mitochondrial dysfunction**—a silent energy crisis happening at the cellular level. Your mitochondria are responsible for creating ATP, the energy currency of the body. But they're fragile. They suffer under oxidative stress, nutritional deficiencies, or environmental toxins. And when they're impaired, every system struggles. You feel it as low energy. Slowed recovery. Weak focus. Even premature aging. And because this damage happens slowly, most people don't notice until the decline feels permanent. But again—this isn't irreversible. The body wants to heal. It just needs the right conditions.

Lastly, there's the psychological load. Many people walk around with constant background stress—overwhelmed by to-do lists, financial worries, social comparison, or even subtle self-criticism. These emotional weights don't just affect the mind. They send biochemical messages that increase inflammation, weaken immunity, and drain energy. When left unchecked, mental burnout becomes physical burnout.

So why are you still tired, foggy, and inflamed? Not because you haven't tried hard enough. But because your body has been signaling overload—and the world hasn't been listening. The answer isn't to do more, push harder, or chase the next hack. It's to slow down and *rebuild*. Step by step.

Layer by layer. Gently peeling back the triggers, replenishing what's been depleted, and learning to trust the messages your body sends.

This chapter isn't about fear. It's about clarity. When you finally understand why your symptoms persist, you stop blaming yourself—and start working *with* your biology instead of against it. From that place, real healing becomes possible.

And that's where we go next.

# Chapter 2: Misdirection in Modern Medicine

## How Medicine Lost Its Way

Modern medicine has saved countless lives. There is no denying the life-changing power of antibiotics, surgical innovation, or emergency care. In moments of crisis, these interventions can mean the difference between life and death. But somewhere along the way, a system originally built to heal began to drift from its roots. It stopped asking why people were getting sick—and focused almost entirely on how to manage the symptoms once they were.

This shift didn't happen overnight. It was gradual, born from a combination of good intentions, scientific excitement, and profit-driven momentum. At first, the rise of laboratory-based science in the 20th century brought breakthroughs that dazzled the world. Bacteria were identified. Diseases were named. Drugs were synthesized. We could finally see the invisible and fight it directly. It felt like magic—and in many ways, it was.

But with every new discovery, the lens narrowed. The human body became a machine made of parts. Each symptom a separate error code to be suppressed or silenced. The body was no longer treated as a living ecosystem—it was managed like a set of malfunctioning compartments. This reductionist approach, while useful in acute scenarios, proved dangerous when applied to chronic illness. Fatigue wasn't seen as a signal—it was treated as depression. Inflammation was controlled with steroids. Blood pressure was "fixed" with a pill. Every marker became a target to push back into range, rather than a clue to be followed. And as pharmaceutical solutions multiplied, fewer practitioners asked *why* the dysfunction arose in the first place.

Part of this disconnect is cultural. Western medicine, for all its brilliance, emerged from a worldview that tends to separate the mind from the body, the body from the environment, and health from lifestyle. Ancient systems of healing—like Traditional Chinese Medicine or Ayurveda—

always viewed health as the result of balance. They saw emotions, food, sleep, seasons, and community as intimately linked to physiology. Modern medicine largely dismissed those links as unscientific. And in doing so, it lost the ability to see patterns before they become problems. Then came the institutionalization of healthcare. Hospitals grew. Insurance systems solidified. And with them came bureaucracy, time pressure, and standardization. Doctors today are often trained to see more patients in less time, using checklists and diagnostic codes to make fast decisions. It's not their fault. The system rewards speed and efficiency, not inquiry and listening. The average medical visit lasts under 15 minutes. That's barely enough time to hear a story, let alone understand it.

And into that space—between the patient and the provider—stepped something else: the pharmaceutical industry. What began as a necessary partnership evolved into something far more influential. Drug companies started funding medical schools, sponsoring research, and shaping treatment guidelines. They advertised not just to doctors, but directly to patients. Illness became a market. Health, a product. And the deeper causes of suffering were buried under symptom charts and branded prescriptions.

We now live in a strange paradox. Medicine has never had more tools, but chronic illness has never been more widespread. Autoimmunity, depression, anxiety, fatigue, brain fog, metabolic dysfunction—these are not niche issues. They are the new normal. And yet most people walk away from their appointments feeling unseen, unheard, and ultimately unsupported. Because the system wasn't designed to help them heal—it was designed to manage them efficiently.

This isn't a criticism of doctors. Most enter the field with the purest intentions. But they're working inside a structure that often prevents them from practicing true healing. The problem isn't a lack of intelligence. It's a lack of time, depth, and freedom to explore root causes.

In the absence of answers, people are left with labels. They're told they have a syndrome, a disorder, a condition—but no one explains how it developed or what can be done to truly reverse it. Instead, they're offered lifelong prescriptions and told to manage it. This isn't care. It's maintenance. And for many, it becomes a quiet sentence of frustration, fatigue, and unanswered questions.

The real tragedy is how many root causes are identifiable and, in many cases, modifiable. Nutrition, sleep, stress, toxic exposures, gut health, movement, emotional trauma—these factors are not fringe. They are foundational. But most of them are either glossed over or dismissed entirely. There is no billing code for "chronic stress." No prescription for "consistent rest." These invisible forces remain under the radar, while the system focuses its resources on downstream effects.

This narrow view of medicine has also left many practitioners exhausted. Burnout among healthcare professionals is at an all-time high. They entered the field to help people heal, only to find themselves stuck in a reactive model that doesn't allow for real connection. The system doesn't reward curiosity. It doesn't fund exploration into healing protocols that can't be patented or easily monetized. Time and again, natural or lifestyle-based interventions are treated as "alternative," despite overwhelming evidence for their effectiveness.

When outcomes are measured by short-term symptom reduction rather than long-term recovery, we get what we now face: a population more medicated than ever, but not necessarily healthier. And behind this sits an even deeper disconnection—from the body itself. When patients are taught that every symptom is an enemy to be eradicated rather than a message to be understood, they lose trust in their own internal cues. Fatigue is fought with caffeine. Anxiety is numbed. Pain is dulled. The body's wisdom is ignored until it breaks down completely.

Rebuilding that trust—both in the body and in a more holistic vision of medicine—starts with awareness. It starts with seeing clearly how we got here. When medicine became dominated by specialization, each organ was given to a different department. The person became a puzzle, fragmented across disciplines. But healing doesn't happen in fragments. Healing requires integration—between systems of the body, between mind and body, and between the person and their environment.

It also requires humility. We've been conditioned to see science as the only valid lens, but science is a method—not a worldview. It's most powerful when it works alongside human experience, not in opposition to it. The idea that a patient's story, intuition, or lived reality is somehow less valid than a lab result is not only flawed—it's dangerous. True healing honors both: the data and the person, the numbers and the narrative.

To move forward, we must return to what medicine was always meant to be: a sacred relationship between healer and human. One that sees symptoms not as isolated malfunctions but as intelligent signals. One that understands that healing is not linear, and that chronic illness often has roots that are emotional, environmental, and deeply personal.

None of this requires abandoning science or rejecting modern innovation. It requires remembering that the human body is more than chemistry. That health is more than absence of disease. And that the role of medicine is not just to extend life—but to restore the vitality and clarity that make life worth living.

The way back is not mysterious. It begins by asking different questions, by listening more closely, and by giving space for the full picture to emerge. When we do, we may find that medicine hasn't failed—it's simply forgotten what it was originally called to do. And once remembered, it can become a force for true healing again. Not just for the body—but for the entire system that was built to protect it.

# When Doctors Say 'It's in Your Head'

There's a particular moment many people with unexplained symptoms know all too well. It comes after countless appointments, inconclusive tests, and months—sometimes years—of suffering. The doctor leans back, sighs gently, and says something like: *"Your results look normal. Maybe it's stress. Maybe it's psychological."* And with that, the invisible door closes. You walk out feeling dismissed, defective, and more alone than ever.

When a doctor tells you *"it's in your head,"* they may mean it innocently. They might be trying to suggest that emotions or mental health could be playing a role. But for many patients, what they hear is: *"You're imagining it. You're exaggerating. This isn't real."* And in a world where symptoms are already undermining your confidence, that subtle dismissal can land like a punch to the gut.

This phrase has become a modern version of a diagnostic dead end. Instead of admitting, *"We don't know what's going on yet,"* the system often reflexively redirects blame inward. It reframes physical suffering as emotional fragility. And worse, it cuts short the investigation. Once a symptom is labeled psychological, it too often gets pushed into the realm of personal responsibility—as if it's your mindset, your trauma, or your failure to cope that's keeping you sick.

This is not just frustrating. It's dangerous.

Modern science increasingly confirms that many chronic and complex illnesses do not show up clearly on standard labs or imaging. Autoimmune disorders can take years to fully reveal themselves. Gut dysbiosis, low-grade inflammation, mitochondrial dysfunction, hormonal imbalances—these may not appear on routine blood work. Yet they cause very real, often debilitating symptoms. To say it's *"in your head"* is to bypass the possibility that our current tools are simply not advanced—or inclusive—enough to detect what's really happening.

What often follows such a dismissal is a deep internal split. On one side, your body continues to cry out with signals—fatigue, pain, brain fog, digestive issues. On the other, the medical system insists that nothing is wrong. You begin to doubt your own perception. You start questioning whether you're being dramatic, or whether it's all just anxiety. That erosion of self-trust is not just emotionally painful—it disconnects you from your most vital compass: your body's signals.

To be clear, this isn't a rejection of the reality that emotions can affect the body. They absolutely can. Trauma, chronic stress, and unprocessed experiences live in the tissues. But acknowledging that truth should expand the conversation—not end it. If anything, it demands more curiosity, more nuance, and more listening—not a hasty handoff to psychiatry or a prescription for antidepressants.

And while many practitioners genuinely want to help, the current system often limits what they can do. Short appointment times, strict diagnostic checklists, and a lack of training in systems biology make it difficult for even well-meaning doctors to explore complex, multifactorial root causes. So, when the tests don't point to a clear answer, it becomes easier—faster, more insurable—to attribute everything to the mind.

But your symptoms are not imaginary. Your pain is not a narrative flaw. And your body is not confused.

This is where we begin to reclaim the conversation. By understanding how real, physiological issues are routinely misdiagnosed or ignored. By looking at how certain populations—especially women—are disproportionately told their symptoms are psychological. And by revealing the scientific links between the mind and body, not as a way to invalidate symptoms, but to expand our understanding of them.

In fact, one of the most unsettling patterns is how often this dismissal falls along lines of gender, race, and socioeconomic status. Studies have repeatedly shown that women's pain is taken less seriously than men's. Women are more likely to be prescribed sedatives than solutions. People of color face similar dismissal—reporting symptoms that are minimized, ignored, or misattributed. Even within the same clinical setting, bias can shape how suffering is perceived and how urgently it is treated. These aren't isolated anecdotes; they're systemic patterns rooted in deep assumptions about who is "credible," who is "dramatic," and who is "worthy" of full investigation.

And so the phrase "It's in your head" becomes more than a personal frustration. It reflects a deeper failure of a medical system still shaped by outdated hierarchies and blind spots. When doctors default to this reasoning, it often reveals more about the limitations of their tools—and their training—than about the patient in front of them.

The truth is, your body and your mind are not separate. But that doesn't mean all physical pain is psychological. Instead, we must move toward a more integrated understanding of how the body stores stress, how trauma rewires biology, and how systemic dysfunction can manifest in ways that don't show up on conventional scans. A body out of balance doesn't always follow the expected script. But it always tells the truth— if we're willing to listen.

Listening, however, requires time. It requires practitioners who are trained to think beyond reductionist models. It requires systems that reward curiosity and holistic thinking instead of penalizing it. And most of all, it requires giving the patient the benefit of the doubt, not because we want to coddle them, but because doing so is scientifically sound and ethically necessary.

There is a reason people are turning to functional medicine, integrative approaches, and root-cause frameworks. Not because they're chasing magic, but because they're tired of being told their suffering is imaginary. They want answers that connect the dots, not brush them away. They want to be seen and heard, not labeled and dismissed.

The damage caused by the "It's in your head" narrative doesn't stop at the emotional level. It also delays diagnosis. It delays healing. It delays critical interventions that could change the trajectory of a person's life. When someone is told their body is fine—even when it clearly isn't— they often stop seeking help. Or they internalize the message and carry shame on top of symptoms. That combination is devastating.

You deserve a model of health that respects complexity. One that knows a body can be biochemically inflamed, hormonally depleted, neurologically misfiring, and emotionally overwhelmed—*all at once*. You deserve clinicians who understand that lab tests are tools, not oracles. That absence of evidence is not evidence of absence. And that if you're

26

showing up and saying something feels off, you are already doing something brave and right.

So if you've been told "it's in your head," here's what you need to remember: You are not broken. You are not exaggerating. You are not weak. You are navigating a system that often wasn't built for complexity, nuance, or true listening—but you are still allowed to expect those things.

Your symptoms are real. Your experience is valid. And your healing doesn't require anyone else's permission.

It begins by reclaiming your story, your signals, and your truth—because your body has never stopped speaking. The question is whether the system was ever ready to hear it.

## The Pill-for-Everything Problem

Walk into almost any home in the developed world and you'll find them: orange bottles in cabinets, daily pill organizers on kitchen counters, half-finished antibiotic courses tucked into drawers. It's not uncommon for people to be taking three, five, even ten medications daily. There's a pill for reflux, a pill for blood pressure, a pill to sleep, a pill to wake up, and a pill to deal with the side effects of the first three. Somewhere along the way, our culture quietly absorbed the idea that every symptom deserves a medication—and that relief must come from a bottle.

This is the pill-for-everything problem. It's not about blaming people who take medications, many of which save lives. It's about asking why so many are prescribed reflexively, why underlying causes are so rarely addressed, and why long-term health is often sacrificed for short-term suppression of symptoms.

Modern medicine has made remarkable advances, particularly in acute care. If you break a bone, need surgery, or face a life-threatening infection, there's no substitute for what hospitals and pharmaceuticals can do. But when it comes to chronic issues—fatigue, inflammation, digestive disorders, hormonal imbalance, brain fog, anxiety—there's been a quiet failure. And into that vacuum, pills have rushed in.

Instead of asking, "Why is the body doing this?" the system asks, "How can we make it stop?" That logic leads to the prescription pad. It's faster. It fits within a 10-minute appointment. And it gives both the doctor and the patient a sense that something is being done. But what happens when that "something" becomes everything?

Take acid reflux as a simple example. Proton pump inhibitors (PPIs) are handed out like candy for indigestion. But many cases of reflux are not caused by excess stomach acid—they're caused by *too little*. The acid is meant to digest food and trigger proper closure of the lower esophageal sphincter. Without enough acid, digestion falters and the valve relaxes, allowing contents to move upward. PPIs may relieve the burning sensation temporarily, but they worsen the core issue and create nutrient deficiencies over time.

Now multiply that by every system in the body. Anti-anxiety medications for nutrient-deprived, dysregulated nervous systems. Statins for inflammation-driven cholesterol problems. Painkillers for joints that are breaking down due to inflammatory diets and sedentary habits. We've designed a reactive medical culture that intervenes with chemistry before it investigates with curiosity.

There is also an economic structure reinforcing this cycle. Pharmaceutical companies are not incentivized to find root causes. Chronic illness, when managed instead of healed, becomes a recurring customer base. The global pharmaceutical market is worth over a trillion dollars, and much of that revenue depends on repeat prescriptions, not one-time cures. When pills become the frontline—and often the only— tool, the system keeps turning, but patients stay stuck.

It's not just the number of prescriptions that's the problem. It's how early we're taught to rely on them. Headache? Take this. Trouble sleeping? Try that. Children, teens, and adults are trained from an early age to reach outward for answers. What's rarely taught is how to look inward: at food, at stress, at sleep, at the environment, at trauma stored in the body. And when those internal issues are left unresolved, no amount of symptom-masking will restore true health.

Once reliance on pills becomes the norm, something deeper is lost—not just in terms of health, but in terms of self-trust. The body is no longer seen as a complex, intelligent system with patterns and signals. It becomes an unpredictable, malfunctioning machine to be chemically controlled. People begin to doubt their instincts. They stop asking why the headaches return every afternoon or why they can't digest food like they used to. If the pill doesn't fix it, the problem must just be "part of life." Or worse—part of them.

This erodes personal agency. Instead of being participants in their health, individuals are positioned as passive recipients of medical directives. Over time, this shapes behavior. Someone who believes they have no power to influence their condition is less likely to change their diet, examine their habits, or challenge the system's assumptions. They wait for the next prescription, hoping it will be the right one.

And yet, underneath that resignation, there's often a quiet frustration—a sense that something isn't adding up. Why, despite all these pills, do I still feel unwell? Why do I have a diagnosis but no clarity? Why do my labs look "normal" but my life doesn't feel that way?

This dissonance is not imagined. The medical model is extraordinary at managing crises, but deeply limited when it comes to understanding the body as an interconnected whole. The pill-for-everything mindset reinforces fragmentation: each symptom gets its own diagnosis, each diagnosis its own medication. But the body doesn't work in isolated compartments. Gut health affects the brain. Hormones respond to sleep. Inflammation doesn't respect specialty boundaries.

What begins as a symptom can quickly become a cascade. A woman is prescribed birth control for irregular cycles. Years later, she's given antidepressants for mood swings, a PPI for reflux, and then thyroid medication for fatigue. No one connects the dots, and she's left believing her body is broken in multiple ways. But the pattern makes sense when you step back and look at the system that taught her to suppress each signal instead of understanding it.

Breaking this cycle requires more than just reducing pill use. It requires restoring belief in the body's ability to heal—gradually, naturally, and often in ways that aren't instant or pharmaceutical. It means learning that a headache might not need ibuprofen, but hydration, rest, or blood sugar balance. That insomnia might be your nervous system calling for regulation. That pain is not always the enemy—it's often information.

There's also a cultural courage required. Saying "no" to a prescription or asking for time before starting a medication can feel like going against authority. But informed consent means just that: being informed. Knowing the pros, the cons, and the alternatives. Knowing that it's okay to explore lifestyle, nutrition, emotional wellness, and environmental health before jumping into long-term chemical interventions.

This isn't anti-medication. It's anti-reflex. Anti-automatic. It's about putting pause between symptom and solution. It's about asking better questions, even when the answers are less convenient. And it's about acknowledging that real healing doesn't always come in pill form.

The most transformative change happens not when a prescription is filled, but when a person begins to observe their body with new eyes. When patterns are tracked. When nutrition is upgraded. When rest is prioritized. When the body is supported rather than silenced. That's when symptoms become guides, not just problems. That's when healing stops being a prescription and starts being a process—one you're actually part of.

Because the truth is, if pills alone could solve our health crisis, we'd be the healthiest society in history. We're not. And the first step to changing that is daring to rethink what we've been told to swallow.

# Chapter 3: Inflammation and Everyday Toxins

## The Hidden Burden of Chronic Inflammation

Chronic inflammation is one of the most misunderstood—and most widespread—drivers of modern illness. It operates quietly, often invisibly, smoldering below the surface of symptoms that are dismissed as everyday nuisances: joint stiffness, brain fog, fatigue, bloating, skin issues, mood swings. Because it doesn't always scream like acute inflammation—a swollen ankle, a red rash, a burning fever—it often goes unrecognized. But its presence can be just as destructive, and in many cases, far more insidious.

At its core, inflammation is a natural, life-saving process. When the body detects injury or infection, it deploys an immune response designed to contain damage and restore balance. This short-term inflammation is essential. It's why you heal from cuts, recover from the flu, or fight off food poisoning. The problem arises when the inflammatory response doesn't shut off. When it persists long after the original trigger is gone— or when the body mistakes normal tissues and processes as threats.

That's when inflammation becomes chronic. And instead of being a healing mechanism, it turns into a source of harm—slowly damaging cells, disrupting hormone signaling, impairing detoxification, and exhausting the immune system. Over time, this chronic low-grade inflammation becomes a silent backdrop to everything else going wrong in the body. You may not see it, but your body feels it every day.

Research now links chronic inflammation to a staggering array of conditions: cardiovascular disease, type 2 diabetes, autoimmune disorders, Alzheimer's, depression, obesity, and even some cancers. Yet few people experiencing these conditions are told that inflammation may be the common thread. They receive medications for their diagnosis— statins, SSRIs, immunosuppressants—but rarely does anyone go upstream to ask what's fueling the fire beneath it all.

That's because chronic inflammation is not a disease. It doesn't have a code. It's not measured on a standard blood test during your yearly checkup. You might get a vague reference to "elevated markers" like CRP or ESR, but those are often dismissed unless they're dangerously high. What's missed is that even mildly elevated inflammatory markers over time are enough to disrupt your health in very real ways.

And more importantly: chronic inflammation rarely comes from just one source. It's cumulative. It builds from years of processed food, environmental toxins, poor sleep, unchecked stress, hidden infections, and gut imbalances. Each piece might not seem enough to tip the scale on its own. But together, they create a body that's constantly in defense mode—fighting battles it was never meant to fight, and running low on the resources needed to repair.

You might feel it as persistent brain fog that no amount of caffeine lifts. Or an irritable gut that flares up after every meal. Or constant muscle tension, hormonal imbalances, a creeping sense of anxiety, or skin that never fully clears. These are not random quirks. They're signals. Signs that the immune system is on edge, operating in a state of over-vigilance. But here's where it gets especially complex: because chronic inflammation becomes normalized. If you've felt tired and bloated and achy for years, you stop questioning it. You assume it's just age, or stress, or genetics. Maybe you even tried changing your diet once or taking a supplement, and when that didn't fix everything, you gave up. Meanwhile, the inflammation continues, shaping the trajectory of your health, undermining your energy, and increasing your risk of serious disease—all while hiding in plain sight.

Medical systems aren't built to address chronic inflammation at its root. They're designed to identify end-stage conditions—when inflammation has already led to a diagnosable disease. Until that threshold is met, your symptoms may be labeled as "nonspecific," "psychosomatic," or "lifestyle-related." You might leave the office with a prescription for heartburn, or a referral to a specialist, but no real investigation into why your body feels like it's constantly on edge.

The truth is, most chronic inflammation is lifestyle-induced—but not in the simplistic way it's often framed. This isn't about "not exercising enough" or "eating too much sugar" in isolation. It's about the cumulative effect of living in a system that makes it incredibly difficult to stay well. A food supply filled with inflammatory oils, additives, and allergens. Air and water laced with endocrine disruptors. Chronic mental stress that your body perceives as physical threat. A sleep-deprived, overstimulated culture that never lets the nervous system unwind.

These constant signals of danger don't just affect your brain—they activate your immune system. They alter your microbiome. They cause intestinal permeability, which allows bacterial fragments and undigested food particles to enter the bloodstream, triggering further immune activation. This isn't fringe science—it's well-documented. And yet, few doctors are trained to connect these dots in clinical practice.

You don't fix chronic inflammation with a single supplement or anti-inflammatory drug. Those may offer short-term relief, but they're not the solution. Addressing inflammation requires peeling back layers—removing irritants, healing the gut, restoring nutrient levels, regulating the stress response, and creating conditions in which the body no longer perceives a constant threat.

And this process isn't fast. Because chronic inflammation didn't appear overnight, it won't disappear overnight either. It's the result of long-term imbalance, and it requires a long-term recalibration. But the payoff is enormous: not just the absence of disease, but the return of vitality, mental clarity, emotional steadiness, and physical ease that many people haven't felt in years.

Still, there's another layer to this that rarely gets discussed: the emotional toll of chronic inflammation. When your body is constantly inflamed, it's not just your joints or digestion that suffer. Your brain does too. Inflammation affects neurotransmitters. It distorts perception. It lowers your threshold for stress and disrupts your sense of safety. That lingering irritability or hopelessness might not be a psychological flaw—it could be a biological fire that hasn't been put out.

And that emotional weight often leads people to self-blame. You wonder why you can't "just feel better." You assume it's weakness, or lack of willpower, or some invisible flaw. But in reality, you're carrying a burden that no one has taught you how to see, let alone release. The first step is recognizing that it's real—and that you're not imagining it, exaggerating it, or overreacting. You're experiencing something your body is desperately trying to communicate.

When you begin to understand chronic inflammation as the common thread behind so much dysfunction—physical, emotional, and cognitive—it becomes easier to stop chasing isolated symptoms and start asking better questions. What is keeping my body inflamed? What patterns, habits, exposures, or beliefs are keeping me stuck in this cycle? And from that place, healing becomes possible. Not in the form of a miracle cure or a rigid protocol, but through the slow, empowering process of reconnecting with your body and supporting the systems that keep it in balance. Chronic inflammation may be hidden, but once revealed, it offers a powerful roadmap—not just for avoiding disease, but for reclaiming the vibrant health that's been muted for far too long.

# The Chemicals in Your Kitchen

Open your pantry or fridge, and you might think you're looking at food. But much of what fills the average kitchen today barely fits that description. Behind the friendly packaging, marketing buzzwords, and long shelf life lies a hidden layer of chemicals — additives, preservatives, synthetic flavors, and industrial compounds — that your body never evolved to process. And for millions of people, this invisible layer is contributing to a silent erosion of health.

The rise of modern convenience foods has reshaped not only how we eat, but what we eat. What used to be a handful of recognizable ingredients has now become a chemistry experiment. In your cereal box, there may be butylated hydroxytoluene (BHT), a petroleum-derived preservative. In your "natural" flavored yogurt, synthetic colorings and artificial sweeteners. In your non-stick pan, residues of perfluorinated compounds that don't break down in your body—or in nature—for decades.

The average consumer is exposed to thousands of these substances every single day, often without knowing it. And while regulators often claim that the small doses are "safe," what they rarely account for is the **cumulative effect**. These aren't isolated exposures. They're repeated, daily, layered on top of each other and compounded by similar chemicals in your shampoo, your tap water, your couch cushions, and your takeout containers.

One of the most concerning classes of chemicals hiding in your kitchen is endocrine disruptors. These substances—like BPA, phthalates, and certain pesticides—interfere with your body's hormonal systems. They can mimic estrogen, block receptors, and throw off the delicate balance that governs everything from metabolism to mood to reproductive health. And they're not just in plastic water bottles. They're in food packaging, in cling wrap, and even in the ink printed on your favorite snack bag.

Another common offender? Ultra-processed emulsifiers and thickeners. Ingredients like polysorbate 80 and carboxymethylcellulose are used to stabilize texture and extend shelf life in everything from ice cream to low-fat salad dressings. But research has shown they can disrupt the gut microbiome, erode the intestinal lining, and promote inflammation—conditions that can lay the groundwork for autoimmunity, obesity, and neurological dysfunction.

Even items marketed as healthy aren't always safe. That oat milk you love may contain synthetic gums and seed oils that quietly fuel inflammation. That "whole grain" frozen dinner might include preservatives banned in other countries. The illusion of safety is powerful, especially when the packaging is covered in claims like "all natural," "no added sugar," or "non-GMO." But these labels are often marketing tactics, not health guarantees.

And it's not just about what's inside the food—it's also about how it's cooked and stored. Non-stick cookware can release toxic fumes at high temperatures. Aluminum foil can leach into acidic or salty foods. Plastic containers—especially when microwaved—can transfer hormone-altering chemicals into your leftovers. Even the water you boil your pasta in may contain residues from agricultural runoff or decaying municipal pipes.

The deeper truth is this: many of the chemicals in your kitchen were never truly tested for long-term safety in humans. They were grandfathered into the food system decades ago, or approved based on outdated or industry-funded studies. The burden of proof has rarely been on manufacturers to prove safety—it's fallen on researchers, whistleblowers, and sick consumers to prove harm. And by the time that harm is acknowledged, it's often too late.

Yet most people still operate under the assumption that "if it's sold in stores, it must be safe." It's a comforting belief, but a dangerous one. Because the agencies responsible for protecting public health are often underfunded, politically influenced, or riddled with industry ties. And the result is a modern food environment where the convenience of chemical-laced products often outweighs the long-term cost to human health.

Children are among the most vulnerable. Their developing bodies are more sensitive to chemical exposure, and yet their diets often include the very foods most loaded with additives—processed snacks, artificial colors, flavor enhancers. Some studies have linked certain food dyes to behavioral issues, including hyperactivity and attention problems. The European Union requires warning labels on foods containing these dyes, while in the U.S., they remain widespread and largely unregulated. It's a silent gamble with our children's biology, traded for visual appeal and product shelf life.

The deeper layer of concern isn't just exposure—it's **bioaccumulation**. Many of these chemicals don't simply pass through the body; they linger. Stored in fat, accumulating over time, subtly interfering with detoxification pathways and endocrine signaling. You can remove a product from your diet, but that doesn't erase the years of exposure already embedded in your tissue. This cumulative load is what researchers now call the "chemical body burden"—the total amount of synthetic compounds residing inside you at any given moment. And while that burden doesn't always produce obvious symptoms immediately, it can weaken the body's resilience, reduce energy, disturb sleep, and increase susceptibility to chronic illness.

The gut is often the first place to show signs of distress. Altered microbiota, compromised gut lining, increased permeability—these are the early cracks in the foundation of health. Over time, these disruptions can trigger immune dysregulation, chronic inflammation, food intolerances, and even neurological symptoms. For many, the cause remains a mystery. But when the kitchen is filled with substances the body doesn't recognize, confusion at the cellular level is inevitable.

And then there's the problem of synergy. Most chemical safety assessments are conducted in isolation. A single preservative, a single artificial color, a single flavoring. But that's not how real life works. Your morning granola bar might contain five different additives, all interacting in ways no one has tested. Your lunch, dinner, snacks, and drinks stack even more. No agency regulates the combined impact of daily exposure to dozens of these compounds. And yet, that's exactly what your body is facing—an unregulated chemical cocktail, day after day.

Some people may say, "Well, we've been eating like this for decades and we're still here." But survival isn't the same as thriving. Chronic disease rates have soared. Autoimmune disorders, allergies, metabolic dysfunction, infertility, cognitive decline—they've all increased at alarming rates. And while correlation is not causation, the timeline tracks closely with the rise in food processing and chemical usage. The body was not designed to thrive in this environment, and many of the illnesses we now normalize may be symptoms of a system in conflict with its fuel source.

The most powerful step you can take isn't to become obsessive or afraid—it's to become aware. Awareness leads to choice. And choice leads to change. Start by reading labels with a critical eye. If you don't recognize an ingredient, ask yourself whether your great-grandmother would have called it food. Choose whole, single-ingredient staples as often as possible. Cook with real fats, not industrial oils. Opt for glass over plastic. Filter your water. Small upgrades, when applied consistently, reduce the total burden. Your body notices. It always does.

This isn't about perfection. It's about stacking the odds in your favor. About creating an internal environment that is as clean, resilient, and stable as possible. Because the reality is: you cannot fully control the external world. But you can control what you bring into your home, what you put on your plate, and what you ask your body to process every day. Your kitchen is either a battleground or a sanctuary. And with every ingredient you allow in, you're casting a vote for one or the other.

## Endocrine Disruptors, Plastics, and Everyday Toxins

If there's one hidden force quietly rewiring the human body, it's the endocrine disruptors that have become embedded in our modern environment. Unlike a sudden trauma or infection, these substances work slowly, subtly, and invisibly—yet their impact is profound. They don't break bones or cause visible bruises, but they can hijack hormones, mimic biological signals, and throw finely tuned systems into chaos. And the most unsettling part? You're likely exposed to them daily, in ways so routine you no longer notice.

The endocrine system—responsible for producing and regulating hormones like estrogen, testosterone, cortisol, insulin, and thyroid hormones—is delicate by design. It functions like a symphony, where timing and dosage are everything. When synthetic chemicals mimic or interfere with these natural messengers, the result isn't just confusion at the cellular level; it's dysfunction. That dysfunction may look like fatigue, weight gain, mood disorders, fertility struggles, irregular cycles, early puberty, or chronic inflammation—and in the long term, it raises the risk for hormone-sensitive cancers and metabolic disease.

One of the most well-known offenders is **BPA** (bisphenol A), a chemical originally developed as a synthetic estrogen. It's found in plastic food containers, canned food linings, water bottles, and even thermal receipt paper. Though many products are now labeled "BPA-free," that label often hides a troubling truth: manufacturers may simply substitute BPA with nearly identical compounds like BPS or BPF, which may be just as disruptive—or worse.

And it's not just about plastics. **Phthalates**, a class of chemicals used to soften plastics and bind fragrances, are also endocrine disruptors. They're found in everything from shampoo and deodorant to plastic packaging and takeout containers. These compounds have been linked to lower testosterone levels, reproductive abnormalities, developmental delays, and altered thyroid function. And once again, the exposure is often invisible. It comes from the lotion you rub into your skin, the air freshener you plug into your wall, or the leftovers you heat in the microwave.

Even our furniture, mattresses, and electronics are often coated with **flame retardants**—many of which are endocrine-disrupting chemicals that can leach into dust and accumulate in our bodies. These compounds may take years to break down and are detectable in human breast milk, umbilical cord blood, and household dust. They build up over time, becoming part of the chemical background noise your body has to manage daily.

What makes endocrine disruptors particularly concerning is that they're active in **minute doses**—far below what toxicologists traditionally considered dangerous. That means even small, repeated exposures can create significant biological effects, especially during critical windows of development like gestation, infancy, and puberty. And unlike poisons that kill cells outright, these compounds often act like faulty keys—unlocking the wrong hormonal doors at the wrong time or jamming the right ones shut.

Most regulatory agencies still evaluate chemical safety using outdated models that focus on high-dose toxicity. They often miss the unique danger of low-dose, long-term exposure to hormone-disrupting chemicals. Meanwhile, the burden of proof remains on the public to demonstrate harm, rather than on manufacturers to prove safety.

So where does that leave us?

It leaves us navigating a world where we're expected to trust that what's on the shelves is safe—when in reality, it's often anything but. And while complete avoidance may be impossible, awareness changes the equation. Knowing where these disruptors hide allows you to start making different choices, choices that protect your body's natural rhythms instead of undermining them.

One of the most powerful steps is rethinking your relationship with plastic. It's not just about ditching plastic water bottles—although that's a good place to start—it's about recognizing how often heat, oil, and acid interact with plastic in everyday settings. Heating leftovers in plastic containers, using plastic wrap on hot food, or drinking coffee from plastic-lined lids all increase your intake of microplastics and their accompanying chemical hitchhikers. Replacing them with glass, stainless steel, or ceramic can quietly but meaningfully reduce your toxic load.

Personal care is another major source of exposure. Many mainstream products contain an unregulated cocktail of endocrine-disrupting chemicals hidden under vague terms like "fragrance" or "parfum." These formulations are often proprietary, meaning companies aren't required to disclose what's in them. Swapping to cleaner, fragrance-free alternatives may feel small, but it's cumulative decisions like these that begin to shift your inner chemistry back toward balance.

Food packaging is just as critical. Even "healthy" convenience foods—like pre-cut vegetables, frozen dinners, or salad mixes—often come wrapped in layers of plastic. Canned goods still rely on linings that may contain BPA analogues. Choosing fresh, unpackaged, or glass-stored items when possible can reduce your ingestion of hormone-disrupting residues that leach into food over time.

It's also worth examining what lingers in the air and dust of your home. Vacuuming with a HEPA filter, regularly dusting with a damp cloth, and ventilating living spaces can all reduce your exposure to flame retardants, phthalates, and other compounds that settle into carpets, upholstery, and electronics. You don't have to live in a bubble, but you can take back some control over what your body is forced to detox daily.

What's striking is how many of these toxins remain legal despite mounting evidence of harm. In the United States, the burden to prove a chemical dangerous often rests on long-term epidemiological studies—while the chemical remains in circulation for decades. The Toxic Substances Control Act, meant to regulate industrial chemicals, has historically allowed thousands of substances onto the market without thorough safety testing. And even when action is taken, it's typically slow, industry-lobbied, and partial.

Meanwhile, Europe and other countries have moved more proactively to regulate certain classes of endocrine disruptors, reflecting a broader cultural willingness to prioritize precaution over convenience. But even there, gaps remain. The reality is globalized commerce and inconsistent regulations mean exposure is still widespread, even across borders.

In the end, understanding endocrine disruptors isn't about living in fear—it's about living informed. It's about choosing materials, products, and behaviors that support your hormonal health instead of undermining it. It's about realizing that your skin, your lungs, your gut—they're all permeable interfaces between you and the world. And that means you get to choose what passes through them.

This is not about perfection. It's about protection. You can't detox your way out of daily exposure if the source isn't addressed. You can't supplement your way around a disrupted system if you're still soaking in the root cause. But you can shift your daily baseline. You can lower your body's toxic burden and give your endocrine system room to recalibrate. And in doing so, you may notice subtle yet profound changes—more stable energy, sharper focus, better sleep, fewer mood swings. These shifts aren't always dramatic, but they are meaningful. They are signs that your body, freed from the constant interference of synthetic intruders, is finally beginning to speak in its own voice again.

# Chapter 4: Gut Instincts—What You've Been Missing

## What Your Gut Is Really Responsible For

We've been taught to think of the gut in terms of digestion alone—food in, waste out. But this is a dangerously outdated framework. Your gut is not just a mechanical tube that processes meals. It is a complex, semi-autonomous ecosystem that influences nearly every system in your body, including your brain, immune system, metabolism, and even your emotional state. If you're feeling chronically tired, inflamed, anxious, foggy, or bloated, the story very often begins—not ends—in your gut.

Inside your gastrointestinal tract, especially in the colon, lives a vast community of bacteria, fungi, viruses, and other microbes—known collectively as the gut microbiome. These organisms are not invaders. In a healthy state, they are collaborators, performing essential tasks your body cannot do alone. They help break down complex fibers, synthesize vitamins like B12 and K2, regulate inflammation, and train your immune system to distinguish between friend and foe.

But here's where things get even more interesting. Your gut and your brain are in constant, two-way communication via the vagus nerve, a kind of information superhighway that transmits chemical and electrical signals between the two. This relationship is so profound that researchers have started referring to the gut as the "second brain." It doesn't just respond to your mental state—it contributes to it. Around 90% of your body's serotonin, the so-called "feel-good" neurotransmitter, is produced in the gut. Dopamine, GABA, and other mood-regulating chemicals also rely on microbial activity for proper balance.

So if your microbiome is out of balance—if it's been disrupted by antibiotics, stress, processed foods, or hidden infections—it doesn't just affect your digestion. It can change how you think, how you feel, and how your body responds to everyday challenges. Anxiety, depression, fatigue, even autoimmune flares—these can all be downstream consequences of an imbalanced gut.

But the gut's role goes beyond even that. It's also one of your body's primary gatekeepers. The lining of the small intestine is only a single cell layer thick—a delicate barrier tasked with deciding what gets absorbed into your bloodstream and what stays out. When this barrier is intact, it functions like a security system, allowing nutrients to pass through while keeping pathogens and toxins at bay. But when the barrier becomes damaged—a condition often referred to as "leaky gut"—the system breaks down.

Undigested food particles, bacterial fragments, and inflammatory molecules can escape into circulation, triggering immune responses that confuse and overload the body. Over time, this can lead to widespread, low-grade inflammation—a root cause behind many modern chronic conditions, from joint pain to brain fog to skin issues.

And yet, this crucial organ system is rarely examined unless you present with overt digestive complaints. Even then, the conventional approach focuses on suppressing symptoms rather than restoring function. Antacids for reflux. Laxatives for constipation. Antibiotics for infections. Few of these address the terrain of the gut itself. Few ask: what caused this imbalance to begin with?

We've inherited a model of medicine that views the body in disconnected parts. But your gut doesn't work in isolation. Its health influences—and is influenced by—your stress levels, your sleep, your food choices, and your exposure to environmental toxins. Every bite you eat, every emotion you suppress, every antibiotic you take without supporting your microbial allies—it all leaves a fingerprint on your gut.

This internal ecosystem thrives on diversity, yet modern life works against it. Diets high in sugar and ultra-processed foods fuel the growth of aggressive, inflammatory microbes while starving the beneficial ones. Chronic stress alters gut motility and reduces protective secretions, making the intestinal lining more vulnerable. Pesticide residues, alcohol, artificial additives, and even over-sanitization contribute to the slow erosion of microbial balance and gut barrier function.

The impact doesn't stop in the intestines. When microbial diversity shrinks and the gut lining weakens, the ripple effects reach far beyond digestion. The immune system—of which nearly 70% is concentrated in gut-associated lymphoid tissue—enters a state of hypervigilance. It starts overreacting to harmless proteins, contributing to the rise in food intolerances and autoimmune conditions. Meanwhile, the constant drip of low-level inflammation burdens the liver, slows cellular repair, and subtly rewires the brain's perception of safety, reinforcing anxiety, mood swings, and fatigue.

What's often labeled as "normal aging" or "stress" is frequently the outward expression of this internal breakdown. The body becomes less resilient not because time has passed, but because the foundational systems sustaining health—like the gut—have been quietly deteriorating. And without an intact gut lining and a balanced microbiome, it becomes nearly impossible to fully absorb nutrients, no matter how healthy your diet looks on paper.

To begin reversing this, the gut must be treated not as a passive organ, but as a dynamic, responsive environment—one that needs to be rebuilt, supported, and protected. That starts with removing the common irritants: processed food, excess alcohol, synthetic additives, and chronic stressors. But removal alone isn't enough. You also need to reintroduce what's been missing: fiber-rich plants, fermented foods, prebiotics, and rest. Reintroduce connection with your meals, with hunger cues, with slowing down enough to chew and digest.

Equally important is restoring gut-brain communication. Practices like breathwork, nervous system regulation, and mindful eating send safety signals to the vagus nerve, activating the "rest and digest" response and allowing the gut to return to its healing rhythm. This isn't alternative medicine—it's fundamental biology, long ignored.

You may also need to address past damage. If you've taken multiple courses of antibiotics or suffered from long-term gut issues, it's possible your microbial diversity has been severely compromised. In those cases, short-term protocols with carefully chosen supplements—like digestive enzymes or specific probiotic strains—may help rebuild the foundation. But these tools are only effective when used alongside a real commitment to lifestyle change.

What makes gut healing both challenging and empowering is that it isn't a quick fix. It requires noticing patterns, tuning in, and becoming your own researcher. It's about moving from suppression to restoration— from masking symptoms to understanding root causes. Most importantly, it's about reclaiming the relationship between you and the intelligence of your body.

People often search for the "one thing" that will solve their fatigue, bloat, or brain fog. But the truth is, the gut doesn't work in isolation, and neither will your healing. The gut is a reflection of how you live: what you feed it, how you move, how you rest, how safe you feel. The real solution isn't found in a miracle food or pill. It's found in rebuilding a terrain where health can once again take root.

Understanding what your gut is truly responsible for changes the conversation from isolated symptoms to systemic insight. This shift is not just biological—it's foundational to restoring sovereignty over your health. When the gut is nourished and supported, your body begins to communicate differently. You become clearer, calmer, more energized. Your resilience returns. And so does your trust in your body's ability to heal.

# The Microbiome and Mental Health

We're finally beginning to understand what ancient systems of medicine intuited long ago: that the gut and the mind are not separate. In recent years, science has uncovered a startling truth—your gut microbiome plays a central role in shaping your thoughts, moods, and mental resilience. It's not just about digestion anymore. The tiny organisms living inside your intestines communicate directly with your brain, and when that communication breaks down, your mental health often suffers.

The term "gut-brain axis" refers to this bidirectional highway between your central nervous system and your enteric nervous system—the vast network of neurons embedded in the walls of your digestive tract. This communication happens through hormones, neurotransmitters, and immune signals, many of which are generated or influenced by your gut microbes. And far from being passive passengers, these microbes act like biochemical factories, producing compounds that either enhance your emotional stability or quietly undermine it.

Take serotonin, for example. Nearly 90% of the body's serotonin—a neurotransmitter critical for mood regulation—is produced in the gut, not the brain. But it's not your own cells that make most of it. It's the bacteria living inside you. These microbes also help produce dopamine, GABA, and short-chain fatty acids, all of which influence how calm, motivated, or emotionally balanced you feel.

When your microbiome is thriving—with a rich, diverse community of bacteria—it can send signals of safety, reduce inflammation, and support a balanced nervous system. But when it's compromised by processed foods, antibiotics, stress, or toxins, that signal becomes scrambled. Inflammation rises, neurotransmitter production falters, and your brain begins interpreting the internal environment as unsafe.

The result? A brain more prone to anxiety, depression, irritability, and brain fog. And here's the catch: most people don't realize it's their gut that's struggling, because the symptoms show up in their head. You might feel short-tempered, unmotivated, or stuck in a loop of negative thoughts—and no one tells you to look at your diet, your digestion, or the invisible ecosystem inside you.

This is especially important for women, who are more likely to experience anxiety and depression and more frequently dismissed with prescriptions that don't address root causes. Hormonal fluctuations, immune sensitivity, and even societal pressure to maintain a "clean" or restricted diet can further disrupt microbial balance, reinforcing the mental load many women carry silently.

Recent studies have begun to explore the use of probiotics—sometimes called "psychobiotics"—to improve mental health outcomes. While not a silver bullet, the results are compelling: certain strains like *Lactobacillus rhamnosus* and *Bifidobacterium longum* have been shown to reduce cortisol, alleviate anxiety, and improve emotional processing. But again, probiotics only work when supported by a lifestyle that promotes microbial diversity: whole foods, fiber, stress reduction, movement, and time in nature.

The gut-brain connection also reframes how we understand trauma. Chronic stress, especially early in life, reshapes the microbiome permanently. Children raised in high-stress environments often have reduced microbial diversity, and this may help explain why they are more vulnerable to mood disorders later on. Trauma doesn't just live in the mind—it lives in the body, and more specifically, in the gut. Healing mental wounds, then, may require addressing the microbial imbalances that trauma left behind.

This perspective offers something powerful: a new entry point for healing. Instead of viewing depression or anxiety as purely chemical imbalances in the brain, we can start seeing them as signals—clues pointing to deeper disruptions that are biological, environmental, and reversible.

This is why some people who've tried every antidepressant and therapy still feel stuck—because the root of their emotional disconnection isn't just psychological. It's biological. When the gut is inflamed, permeable, and out of balance, it constantly sends distress signals that the brain can't ignore. The system becomes locked in a loop of low-grade emergency, and no amount of mindset work can fully override that signal without addressing the source.

The modern diet plays a huge role in this cycle. Ultra-processed foods don't just lack nutrients—they actively damage the gut lining and feed harmful bacteria. Refined sugars and industrial oils fuel the growth of inflammatory microbes that disrupt the gut-brain axis. Artificial sweeteners, preservatives, emulsifiers, and other additives—while technically "safe" by regulatory standards—can disturb microbial communication in subtle but meaningful ways. What's marketed as harmless convenience food becomes a daily assault on the balance of your inner ecosystem.

Equally damaging is the chronic stress most people live under without realizing it. Psychological stress changes the composition of the microbiome, favoring bacteria that thrive in high-stress, inflammatory environments. It's a self-reinforcing cycle: stress harms the gut, and a disrupted gut makes you more sensitive to stress. This is why the same life situation can feel manageable on one day and completely overwhelming the next—depending on what your gut is signaling to your brain.

Sleep, movement, and connection are also major players. Poor sleep quality weakens the gut barrier, reducing resilience and amplifying systemic inflammation. Sedentary lifestyles limit microbial diversity and stagnate circulation. Isolation from others cuts off one of the most ancient and effective regulators of nervous system health—social bonding, which is tightly linked to microbial exchange and emotional regulation.

This might sound like bad news, but in truth, it opens the door to a level of healing that many people have never been offered. If you've ever felt like your emotions didn't match your life circumstances—if you've woken up feeling anxious for no reason, struggled to concentrate, or felt emotionally flat despite "doing everything right"—your body may be trying to tell you that your internal ecosystem needs repair.

The good news is that the microbiome is dynamic. With the right inputs, it can regenerate quickly. In some studies, measurable improvements in gut composition—and mood—occurred within just a few weeks of diet change. Fiber-rich foods, fermented vegetables, resistant starches, prebiotics, and polyphenols act like fertilizer for beneficial bacteria. Real food, eaten consistently and with awareness, becomes mental medicine. And while probiotics can be helpful, they are not a substitute for the foundational work. A capsule can't override a daily diet of gut-disrupting substances or a life lived in chronic stress. Healing your microbiome means living in a way that honors its needs: nourishment, rest, movement, connection, and a slower pace. It means thinking about how you feed not just yourself, but the thousands of species within you that help regulate how you feel.

This shift is radical because it decentralizes the idea that your mind is separate from your body. It moves away from blaming yourself for how you feel, and instead teaches you to investigate the physiological signals shaping your mood. It invites compassion—toward yourself and your biology.

You are not broken. Your sadness, your overwhelm, your lack of clarity—these are not character flaws. They are adaptations, shaped in part by the condition of the invisible world inside you. When you begin to tend to that world, things often shift. You start to feel steadier, clearer, more at ease. The fog lifts—not because you forced it, but because you supported the system that was silently holding you back.

For many, this is the missing piece. And for some, it's the beginning of true mental freedom. Not from suppressing symptoms, but from finally understanding their source—and healing it from the inside out.

## Antibiotics, Food, and the Gut Breakdown

For decades, antibiotics have been hailed as one of the greatest medical breakthroughs in human history—and rightfully so. They've saved countless lives by fighting off infections that once meant certain death. But the story didn't end with their life-saving potential. Over time, antibiotics went from being carefully administered medicine to something far more casual—overprescribed, misunderstood, and, most critically, overused in places most people don't even realize.

What began as a miracle of modern medicine quietly became a slow assault on the microbiome. Every time you take antibiotics, you're not just killing the bacteria that made you sick—you're also killing vast numbers of beneficial microbes that your body depends on. Your gut is home to trillions of organisms that regulate digestion, immunity, inflammation, and even brain chemistry. When that balance is disrupted, the effects ripple far beyond your stomach.

The problem isn't just the antibiotics you've been prescribed by a doctor. It's also the antibiotics you've unknowingly consumed through the food system. In industrial agriculture, antibiotics are routinely fed to livestock—not primarily to treat disease, but to promote faster growth and prevent illness in overcrowded, unsanitary conditions. These antibiotic residues end up in the meat, dairy, and even the water supply, subtly altering our internal ecosystems over time.

The result is a population that is chronically inflamed, metabolically dysregulated, and missing key microbial species necessary for long-term health. And most people have no idea it's happening. You might feel tired for no reason, bloated after meals, or mentally foggy without knowing that your microbiome has been under siege for years. You might crave sugar constantly, feel mood swings you can't explain, or experience unexplained food sensitivities—all signs of a gut environment that's out of sync with its natural design.

Worse still, repeated antibiotic exposure—whether from prescriptions or food—can lead to antibiotic resistance, meaning the drugs are less effective when you truly need them. It's a vicious cycle. The more we overuse them, the less they work, and the more damage we do to the very systems meant to protect us.

Many people also don't realize how long it takes for the gut to recover after a round of antibiotics. Some studies suggest that even a single course can disrupt the microbiome for months. And when the diet remains poor—lacking fiber, rich in processed foods—the gut doesn't fully bounce back. Instead, opportunistic microbes take over, producing inflammatory compounds and crowding out beneficial bacteria. This microbial imbalance, known as dysbiosis, can manifest in symptoms that are easy to dismiss: gas, bloating, constipation, mild depression, skin issues, poor concentration. But over time, those small signs become the roots of chronic illness.

Food becomes a key player in either healing or worsening the damage. Unfortunately, the modern diet often fuels the breakdown rather than reversing it. Refined grains, industrial oils, excessive sugar, artificial ingredients—all of these feed the wrong microbes and starve the right ones. This doesn't just affect digestion—it affects your entire system. A compromised gut barrier can allow endotoxins to enter the bloodstream, triggering an immune response that creates low-grade systemic inflammation. That inflammation is now linked to virtually every major chronic illness, from autoimmune diseases to metabolic syndrome to neurodegeneration.

At this point, it's easy to feel overwhelmed. The scale of the problem is massive, and most people are living in the middle of it, unknowingly feeding the very system that's eroding their health. But knowledge is the beginning of empowerment. When you understand how antibiotics and food interact with your body, you can start to make choices that interrupt the cycle.

Let's now look at what it actually takes to restore the gut after damage, and how to use food strategically—not just to nourish, but to rebuild.

Rebuilding the gut begins with removing the inputs that keep harming it. That means avoiding unnecessary antibiotics—not just prescriptions, but also those hidden in food. Choosing meat and dairy from animals raised without antibiotics isn't a trend—it's a step toward protecting your own internal ecosystem. Even better, shifting toward plant-forward meals rich in diverse, whole foods gives the gut a break from inflammatory and antibiotic-laden products while feeding the microbes that matter.

But it's not just about what you take out—it's about what you put in. Fiber becomes a foundational tool. Not just the kind found in fortified cereals, but real, fermentable fibers from vegetables, legumes, nuts, seeds, and whole fruits. These act as prebiotics—fuel for beneficial bacteria. Without that fuel, even a well-intentioned probiotic won't stick. Many people don't realize that swallowing capsules full of live bacteria doesn't do much if the terrain isn't right. The gut environment needs to be hospitable—rich in the kinds of fibers, polyphenols, and compounds that allow good microbes to thrive.

Fermented foods also help. They're not just trendy—they're ancient tools for microbial balance. Sauerkraut, kimchi, kefir, miso, real yogurt—when made properly, these are living foods that deliver diverse species of microbes to the gut and help restore what was lost. They don't act like a pharmaceutical fix; they act like reinforcements to a struggling ecosystem.

Still, many people try all the "right" things and see little improvement. That's often because the damage is deeper. The gut lining may be compromised—tiny junctions meant to keep pathogens and toxins out of the bloodstream may have loosened, allowing things to pass through that shouldn't. This is often referred to as "leaky gut," and while some dismiss the term, the physiological reality is real. It creates a steady trickle of inflammation, burdening the immune system and triggering systemic effects—everything from autoimmune flares to brain fog to persistent skin issues.

To rebuild the gut lining, nutrients like glutamine, zinc, and collagen can help, but the foundation is always food. Anti-inflammatory fats like those in wild fish, flax, and olive oil reduce damage. Colorful vegetables and berries provide antioxidants to neutralize oxidative stress. Bone broths and properly prepared legumes offer soothing, restorative nutrients. And timing matters too. Giving the gut rest through overnight fasting windows—12 to 14 hours without food—allows it to clean house and reset.

Stress, often underestimated, is another key player. The gut and brain are deeply connected—if your nervous system is constantly in a state of fight-or-flight, the gut won't function properly, no matter how clean your diet is. Practices that regulate the nervous system—breathwork, walking, nature, slow meals, mindfulness—become gut repair tools as much as anything on your plate. Healing is not just chemical; it's energetic and emotional, too.

Even after all this, progress isn't always linear. Setbacks happen. Flare-ups return. But the body remembers what balance feels like. With consistent inputs, it moves toward homeostasis. You don't need perfection—you need persistence. You need the awareness to recognize what harms you and the courage to change what's been considered "normal" for too long.

Because the truth is, this gut breakdown isn't just about biology—it's about culture. About a society that prizes speed over nourishment, industrial convenience over health, and symptom suppression over root cause resolution. Rebuilding your gut is a quiet act of resistance. It's a refusal to keep feeding the system that made you sick in the first place.

And as the gut restores, everything begins to shift. Energy stabilizes. Mood lifts. Immunity strengthens. Food becomes pleasure again instead of fear. This isn't just about digestion—it's about reclaiming a sense of power over your body. It's the beginning of a deeper health reset that touches every system, every organ, every part of who you are.

It starts in the gut. But it doesn't end there.

# Chapter 5: The Hormone Crash

## The Hormonal Havoc of Modern Life

Hormones don't just regulate reproduction—they orchestrate nearly every system in the body. Energy, sleep, metabolism, mood, libido, stress response, appetite, immune function, and even memory are all governed by the ebb and flow of hormonal signals. When these messengers are in balance, the body operates like a finely tuned machine. But when modern life throws that system off—as it so often does—the consequences ripple through every corner of health.

In many ways, we're living in a hormonal minefield. The delicate endocrine system wasn't designed to cope with the constant barrage of stress, synthetic chemicals, disrupted circadian rhythms, blood sugar spikes, and poor-quality sleep that define the modern experience. What results is hormonal chaos—subtle at first, but progressively harder to ignore. Fatigue that doesn't lift, sleep that never feels restorative, unexplained weight gain, anxiety without clear cause, irritability, brain fog, and the persistent sense that something just isn't right.

It's easy to write these off as signs of aging, personality, or busyness. But underneath, the root often lies in disrupted hormonal communication. Cortisol—the body's primary stress hormone—was designed for acute danger, not chronic emails, traffic, and doom-scrolling. When cortisol is chronically elevated, it throws off everything else. It suppresses thyroid function, disrupts insulin signaling, and increases abdominal fat storage, especially the kind most linked to inflammation and disease.

Insulin, the hormone that regulates blood sugar, gets pushed to its limits by the way many people eat—refined carbs, constant snacking, sweetened beverages, and processed food devoid of fiber or nutrients. When insulin is always high, cells stop responding to it efficiently, leading to insulin resistance, blood sugar instability, and eventually the path toward type 2 diabetes and metabolic syndrome. But even before that point, the hormonal fallout can already be felt—energy crashes, sugar cravings, brain fog, and mood swings that feel impossible to control.

Sex hormones like estrogen, progesterone, and testosterone are also profoundly influenced by lifestyle. For women, chronic stress can rob the body of progesterone in favor of making more cortisol—a phenomenon sometimes referred to as the "pregnenolone steal." The result? Cycles become irregular, PMS worsens, and symptoms like anxiety, sleep disruption, or low libido creep in. For men, poor sleep, excess alcohol, belly fat, and endocrine-disrupting chemicals all chip away at testosterone levels—reducing drive, energy, and focus.

Thyroid function, too, is incredibly sensitive to this hormonal storm. The thyroid controls the pace of metabolism, but it requires safety signals from the body to function optimally. Chronic stress, inflammation, nutrient deficiencies (especially iodine, selenium, and zinc), and gut issues can all slow the thyroid down. The result is a body that feels sluggish no matter how many hours you sleep or how much coffee you drink. Many people go undiagnosed for years because their symptoms don't show up clearly on basic lab tests, but the internal dysfunction is already affecting everything from digestion to cognition to immune response.

The environment adds fuel to the fire. Endocrine disruptors—found in plastics, pesticides, personal care products, non-stick cookware, and even receipts—mimic hormones in the body and interfere with normal signaling. They don't just confuse the body; they can actively downregulate or upregulate real hormone production. For example, BPA, a common chemical found in many plastics, can mimic estrogen and throw off hormonal balance in both men and women. Phthalates, parabens, and other synthetic chemicals have similar effects. And exposure isn't occasional—it's daily, cumulative, and often invisible.

The cumulative result of all these modern influences is a body constantly playing hormonal whack-a-mole—trying to stay in balance while the inputs keep pushing it further off center. Most people don't realize their symptoms—physical or emotional—could be traced back to these internal messengers. But once that connection is made, it becomes impossible to unsee. Hormonal health isn't a fringe topic—it's the foundation of vitality.

Once hormonal imbalance sets in, the body often tries to compensate. That compensation, though, can trigger secondary issues—sluggish digestion, lowered immunity, constant fatigue, irregular sleep cycles, skin issues, and mood dysregulation. Instead of being treated as interconnected symptoms, they're usually approached in isolation. A pill for sleep. A pill for mood. A stimulant for energy. But the underlying endocrine dysfunction remains untouched.

One of the most misunderstood aspects of this hormonal spiral is how it affects women throughout their monthly cycle and across life stages. Symptoms like irritability, bloating, breast tenderness, migraines, and sleep disruption are normalized or minimized, yet they often reflect estrogen dominance, low progesterone, or disrupted cortisol patterns. Perimenopause—once considered a smooth and natural transition—has become for many women a time of upheaval. With hormones already on edge from environmental stressors, the drop in estrogen and progesterone only intensifies symptoms. Instead of seeing this as a sign to recalibrate, conventional medicine often labels it as anxiety, depression, or aging—and responds with antidepressants or hormone blockers.

For men, the gradual but steady decline in testosterone is often written off as aging, but it's happening earlier and more rapidly than in previous generations. Low energy, reduced motivation, loss of muscle mass, brain fog, and increased fat storage aren't just midlife problems—they're consequences of a system out of sync. Add in poor sleep, alcohol, processed foods, and constant screen exposure at night (which disrupts melatonin and indirectly testosterone), and it becomes a perfect storm.

Sleep itself is a hormonal process, governed by the interplay of melatonin, cortisol, and insulin. Poor sleep throws those rhythms off, and those disrupted rhythms worsen sleep in return. It's a self-perpetuating loop. The same goes for appetite and satiety. Hormones like leptin, ghrelin, and insulin regulate how hungry we feel, how satisfied we get from food, and where our body stores fat. When these signals are dysregulated, it leads to cravings, overeating, and weight gain—often in spite of conscious efforts to eat less.

And underneath it all, inflammation plays a silent role. Inflammatory signals can suppress thyroid function, interfere with insulin sensitivity, and disrupt sex hormone production. This is why someone dealing with chronic joint pain, gut issues, or an autoimmune condition may simultaneously struggle with fatigue, mood swings, or irregular cycles. It's not separate. It's systemic.

The tragedy is that many people spend years looking for answers in the wrong places—trying diet after diet, blaming themselves for lack of willpower, accepting that feeling unwell is just their "normal." They often hear that their labs are "fine" or that their symptoms are vague. But a normal lab result doesn't mean optimal health. It just means falling within a wide reference range that doesn't account for how you actually feel.

True hormonal health requires a shift in thinking. It's not about forcing balance with synthetic hormones or silencing symptoms with medications. It's about restoring the conditions that allow the body to regulate itself. That includes quality sleep, blood sugar stability, stress reduction, exposure to natural light, movement, nutrient density, gut health, and minimizing toxic exposures. None of it is a quick fix. But it works—because it's working with the body, not against it.

Most people don't need more willpower. They need restoration. When hormones begin to normalize, the fog lifts. Energy returns. Sleep deepens. Emotions stabilize. The body stops fighting itself and starts to heal. That's the promise of understanding what hormonal havoc really means—and what reversing it can look like.

This isn't fringe wellness—it's foundational biology. And recognizing that gives people their power back. Not in theory. Not someday. But now. Because when you change the signals you send your body, the response is often faster and more profound than anyone told you to expect.

## Cortisol, Fatigue, and the Stress Spiral

If there's one hormone that perfectly encapsulates the pace, pressure, and exhaustion of modern life, it's cortisol. Known as the "stress hormone," cortisol is produced by the adrenal glands and plays a critical role in our daily rhythm, energy levels, immune function, metabolism, and even memory. At healthy levels, cortisol follows a natural arc—it peaks in the morning to wake us up and gradually tapers off through the day to allow restful sleep. This rhythm is essential for feeling alert during the day and winding down at night.

But in our chronically stressed world, this pattern is rarely intact. The problem isn't cortisol itself—it's how often and how long it's being triggered. Cortisol is designed for acute stress, like escaping danger. It was never meant to be pumped out constantly in response to deadlines, arguments, bills, lack of sleep, and the silent pressure of never feeling "enough." When that happens, cortisol goes from being helpful to being harmful. And the body, over time, starts to pay the price.

The first signs are usually subtle—an afternoon energy crash, trouble falling asleep even when tired, or waking up wired in the middle of the night. These are signs that cortisol rhythms are no longer aligned with the body's natural needs. As the disruption continues, it often evolves into persistent fatigue, brain fog, irritability, increased belly fat, and reliance on caffeine to function. Many people assume these are just signs of aging or a busy life. In truth, they're symptoms of a deeper physiological imbalance.

The stress spiral begins when cortisol production becomes dysregulated. Initially, the body may overproduce cortisol in response to nonstop demands. This phase can feel deceptively productive—people feel energized, wired, even euphoric under pressure. But underneath, the system is burning through nutrients, taxing the adrenals, and overriding the need for recovery. Over time, the body shifts into the opposite problem: cortisol starts to drop too low. The result? A profound, bone-deep fatigue that sleep doesn't fix.

This state—often referred to as "adrenal fatigue" or more accurately, HPA axis dysfunction—is not recognized as a formal medical diagnosis, but its effects are very real. It occurs when the hypothalamus, pituitary gland, and adrenal glands (the HPA axis) stop responding to stress properly. The signals get scrambled. Cortisol output flattens out, leading to a muted response to stress during the day and poor energy production. People wake up feeling exhausted and stay that way regardless of how much they rest.

Adding to the problem, modern stress is rarely "fight or flight" anymore—it's chronic and ambient. It comes from juggling multiple roles, financial pressure, information overload, emotional disconnection, and an always-on digital world that never lets the brain power down. The body can't tell the difference between a real threat and an inbox full of urgent messages. To cortisol, it all feels like danger. And that constant alert status keeps the nervous system locked in a state of low-grade tension.

At the same time, cortisol and insulin are deeply intertwined. When cortisol is elevated, it can make the body more insulin resistant, driving blood sugar spikes and crashes. This leads to cravings, especially for sugar and refined carbs, which then reinforce the stress response even more. It's a vicious cycle: stress raises cortisol, cortisol disrupts blood sugar, unstable blood sugar creates more stress, and the loop keeps feeding itself.

This is where the fatigue becomes more than just feeling tired—it becomes a full-body energy collapse. The kind where no amount of sleep feels refreshing, and motivation disappears. Where even small tasks feel overwhelming. This isn't laziness or lack of willpower. It's the body asking for help.

When this chronic output and eventual depletion of cortisol go unchecked, it starts to erode the body's foundational systems. Digestion slows down, the immune system weakens, and the repair mechanisms that normally restore tissue, regulate hormones, and keep inflammation in check begin to falter. Over time, the symptoms shift from simple exhaustion to more complex dysfunction—frequent colds, worsening allergies, digestive issues, and hormonal imbalances that show up as irregular cycles, low libido, or weight gain despite unchanged habits.

Sleep suffers in tandem. Cortisol should be lowest at night, allowing melatonin to rise and signal deep rest. But in many people, that pattern is reversed—cortisol spikes in the evening, keeping the mind racing long after the body wants to shut down. Even if sleep comes, it's light and fragmented, never reaching the restorative depth needed to heal the nervous system. This only reinforces the cycle: the body wakes unrested, demands caffeine or sugar to cope, and ends the day once again in a state of wired fatigue.

Eventually, the emotional layer begins to crack. Chronic dysregulation of cortisol is linked to increased anxiety, depression, irritability, and a sense of emotional numbness. The nervous system, overwhelmed for too long, loses its resilience. Things that once felt manageable start to feel unbearable. The inner flame dims—not because of weakness, but because the body is trying to conserve the little energy it has left. And in this state, people often begin to believe something is deeply wrong with them, when in truth, the system has just been pushed too far for too long.

This is where conventional medicine often falls short. Lab results may come back "normal," because standard cortisol tests often miss the nuances of dysfunction. A single snapshot doesn't capture the diurnal rhythm—the rise and fall across the day—that reveals the real picture. Many patients are told they're fine, or worse, that their fatigue is "psychological." But anyone who has lived in this state knows it's not in their head. It's in every cell of their body.

Restoring balance begins with removing the constant demand. This isn't about quitting life or avoiding responsibilities—it's about creating moments where the body feels safe again. That might mean reducing caffeine, setting boundaries with technology, protecting sleep like it's sacred, or simply taking five minutes each day to breathe deeply and do nothing. These shifts may seem small, but to a body starved for calm, they're signals of safety. And safety is the prerequisite for healing.

Food plays a crucial role too. Stabilizing blood sugar with protein-rich meals, whole foods, and healthy fats reduces cortisol surges and supports the adrenal glands. Replenishing depleted nutrients—especially magnesium, B vitamins, and vitamin C—helps rebuild the pathways that regulate stress. Movement, when gentle and supportive rather than punishing, tells the body it's not under threat. Even walking in nature can help reset cortisol rhythms and return the nervous system to baseline.

But perhaps the most important step is to shift the relationship with stress itself. So many people are caught in the belief that they must earn rest, prove their worth, or push through no matter what. These internalized patterns are often more damaging than the external stressors themselves. Learning to recognize the signs of depletion early, to pause before collapse, and to honor the body's signals instead of overriding them—that's where real healing begins.

Cortisol is not the enemy. It's a messenger. And when it's out of balance, it's not a failure—it's feedback. The body is always trying to adapt, to survive, to protect you. When it whispers that it's had enough, the bravest thing you can do is listen. Because on the other side of that spiral is not just relief—it's restoration. And with it, the clarity, energy, and stability that make life not just manageable again, but meaningful.

# Why Your Thyroid Can't Keep Up

You wake up tired. You drag through the day. Your hands are cold, your skin is dry, your mood is flat. Maybe your hair is thinning, your weight creeping up even though you haven't changed how you eat. And still—your doctor says your thyroid labs are "normal." This is the frustrating reality many people, especially women, face when their thyroid is quietly struggling, even before it crosses the threshold of disease.

The thyroid is a small, butterfly-shaped gland in the neck, but its impact is massive. It regulates your metabolism—how fast or slow your body uses energy. It influences mood, heart rate, digestion, temperature, brain function, and more. When the thyroid slows down, everything else does too. It's not just a matter of energy. It's a full-system slowdown that affects how alive you feel in your body.

So why is this powerful little gland under such pressure today?

One of the most overlooked reasons is stress. Chronic stress doesn't just wear out your nerves—it alters your entire endocrine system. When cortisol is constantly elevated, it sends a message to your body that survival—not reproduction, growth, or thriving—is the priority. In that environment, thyroid function is downregulated. The conversion of the storage hormone T4 into the active hormone T3 slows down, and more of it is shunted into an inactive form, reverse T3. The signal gets weaker, even if the raw materials are technically still there.

But stress isn't the only culprit. Nutrient deficiencies are common and often missed. Your thyroid relies on specific nutrients to function—iodine, selenium, zinc, iron, and tyrosine among them. When these are depleted, often due to poor absorption, poor diet, or chronic inflammation, the thyroid doesn't have the raw materials it needs to work properly. Think of it like trying to bake a cake without flour—it doesn't matter how hot the oven is if the ingredients are missing.

Another hidden factor is autoimmunity. Hashimoto's thyroiditis is the most common cause of hypothyroidism in the developed world, and it's an autoimmune condition—meaning the body is attacking its own thyroid tissue. This often develops silently for years before labs show clear signs of dysfunction. And yet, unless antibodies are tested (which many conventional panels don't include), the autoimmune component can go completely undiagnosed. In these cases, replacing thyroid hormone may help symptoms, but it doesn't address the root—why the immune system turned on the thyroid in the first place.

Toxins, too, play a role. Endocrine disruptors found in plastics, personal care products, pesticides, and even some tap water can interfere with thyroid hormone signaling. They can mimic or block hormones at the receptor level, confuse the body's feedback loops, and even damage the gland itself. Over time, the cumulative burden becomes too much.

There's also the issue of the gut. An imbalanced microbiome and increased intestinal permeability ("leaky gut") have been linked to autoimmunity, including Hashimoto's. When the gut barrier breaks down, food particles and bacterial fragments can slip into the bloodstream and trigger immune reactions. If the immune system mistakes thyroid tissue for a foreign invader due to molecular mimicry, it begins a slow attack that erodes function over time.

But perhaps one of the most frustrating parts of thyroid dysfunction today is how often it's dismissed. A standard thyroid panel usually checks just TSH (thyroid stimulating hormone), which is a brain signal—not the actual thyroid hormone levels. TSH can remain within the so-called normal range even when free T3 and free T4 are low or poorly converted. Many people fall into a gray zone: not quite sick enough for a diagnosis, but not well either. And so they're left untreated, unheard, and exhausted.

Instead of being offered deeper testing or nutritional support, many people are told that what they're experiencing is just aging, stress, or depression. They may be given antidepressants, told to exercise more, or simply reassured that "everything looks fine." But symptoms persist, and so does the feeling of not being heard. This dismissal is not only frustrating—it delays the identification of underlying dysfunction and keeps people stuck in a loop of invisible illness.

On a physiological level, even small imbalances in thyroid hormone can have wide-ranging effects. When your cells don't receive adequate

65

thyroid signals, your metabolism slows—not just in terms of weight, but in cellular energy production. Mitochondria, the powerhouses of your cells, become less efficient. This can lead to feelings of fatigue that aren't improved by rest. You don't just feel tired—you feel like you're running on empty, no matter how much sleep you get.

Body temperature regulation may shift subtly, often showing up as cold hands and feet, or a general intolerance to cold weather. Digestion can slow, leading to constipation and bloating. Brain fog creeps in—making it hard to concentrate, recall words, or stay sharp in conversation. Skin becomes dry, nails brittle, hair sheds more than usual. For many, these symptoms accumulate slowly, until they feel like a lesser version of themselves—no obvious illness, just a steady decline.

Even mood is affected. Low thyroid function can contribute to depression and anxiety, not just because of how it makes you feel physically, but due to direct effects on neurotransmitters. Serotonin and dopamine pathways don't function the same in a low-metabolic state. The body starts conserving energy, and the brain can mirror that slowing—leaving you feeling emotionally flat or unable to fully engage with life.

Compounding this is the reality that many people—especially women—are juggling other hormonal imbalances at the same time. Estrogen dominance, perimenopausal shifts, or blood sugar instability can all place additional strain on the thyroid. The body doesn't experience these systems in isolation. When one hormone is off, it often drags others with it. And yet, conventional care typically slices the body into disconnected parts, missing the patterns that tell the real story.

This is why a functional approach to thyroid health looks beyond just numbers. It listens to symptoms, considers the whole picture, and asks deeper questions: Are nutrients being absorbed? Is the gut inflamed? Is stress unresolved? Are toxins accumulating faster than they can be cleared? Are antibodies present, and if so, why?

It also means recognizing that supporting the thyroid isn't always about medication. For some, yes, thyroid hormone replacement is life-changing and necessary. But for many others, the most powerful shift comes from addressing the underlying pressure on the system—supporting the adrenals, replenishing nutrients, healing the gut, removing hidden stressors, and restoring a sense of safety in the body.

Reclaiming thyroid health isn't about chasing perfect labs. It's about returning to a state where your body trusts itself again—where energy flows, where warmth returns to your hands, where your mind clears, and your voice feels strong in the world. It's not a quick fix. But with the right guidance and curiosity, it's possible to reconnect with this core piece of your biology and start feeling like yourself again.

This chapter isn't about alarm. It's about awareness. Your thyroid is trying to keep up in a world that makes it incredibly hard to do so. But when you understand what it needs—and begin clearing the obstacles in its way—you give it the conditions to recover. And in doing that, you give yourself the possibility of a life not ruled by fatigue, fog, or frustration—but one marked by vitality, clarity, and calm.

# Chapter 6: Inflammation's Hidden Toll

## What Inflammation Really Does to You

We've all heard of inflammation—usually in the context of injuries or autoimmune disease—but for most people, it's still a vague concept. A red, swollen ankle. An allergic reaction. A fever. That's inflammation, right? Yes—but that's only the most visible end of the spectrum. The real problem lies in the hidden, chronic kind. The inflammation you don't see. The inflammation that simmers silently in your body, year after year, shaping your health without ever calling attention to itself.

Chronic inflammation doesn't come with bandages or dramatic symptoms. It's the background noise of a modern life—created by processed food, environmental toxins, gut imbalances, emotional stress, poor sleep, overmedication, and more. While acute inflammation is your body's natural way of healing—a short, targeted burst of immune activity to clean up damage or fight off invaders—chronic inflammation is something else entirely. It's the immune system turned on and left running without a clear reason, quietly damaging tissues and organs over time.

And this is where the real danger lies. Because when inflammation becomes chronic, it doesn't just cause discomfort—it lays the foundation for nearly every major disease of our time. Heart disease, Alzheimer's, cancer, diabetes, autoimmune conditions, depression, infertility, even accelerated aging—all of them have a link to chronic, low-grade inflammation. It's not the only factor, but it's a common thread. A slow-burn fire smoldering in the background of your biology. But what exactly is happening when you're inflamed?

Imagine your immune system as a highly trained defense team. When you're injured or sick, it activates, sends white blood cells to the scene, and floods the area with chemical messengers—cytokines, histamines, prostaglandins—to isolate the problem and begin repair. If everything goes well, the damage is contained, the debris is cleared, and the immune system powers down.

But in chronic inflammation, this off-switch gets stuck. The system keeps reacting, even when there's no clear threat. Maybe because there's a leaky gut, and food particles are slipping into the bloodstream. Maybe because you're eating processed seed oils every day. Maybe because you're under so much emotional stress that your body constantly perceives danger. The triggers vary. But the result is the same: your immune system never gets to rest.

This constant state of alert has consequences. Inflammation begins to damage healthy cells, degrade tissues, disrupt hormones, interfere with brain chemistry, and exhaust the body's natural repair systems. You may not feel "sick" in the traditional sense, but symptoms start to appear— low energy, brain fog, joint stiffness, bloating, skin issues, weight gain that doesn't respond to diet, mood swings. They're not just random. They're the language of inflammation.

One of the most overlooked aspects of this process is how inflammation affects your brain. Neuroinflammation—chronic immune activity in the brain—has been linked to depression, anxiety, cognitive decline, and even neurodegenerative diseases. If you've ever felt like your thoughts are heavy or your motivation has vanished without explanation, inflammation could be playing a role. And the worst part? Most conventional evaluations won't catch it, because inflammatory symptoms rarely show up in basic blood tests unless the situation is already advanced.

Nowhere is this more evident than in the gut. The intestinal lining is only one cell thick—a fragile barrier that, when compromised, allows unwanted particles into the bloodstream. This is what's commonly referred to as "leaky gut." And once that barrier is broken, the immune system starts reacting to everything: food, bacteria, toxins, even your own tissue. Over time, this chronic immune activation can lead to food sensitivities, skin conditions, fatigue, joint pain, and autoimmune disease. All quietly building from inflammation that started in the gut.

When the immune system is constantly activated, it also begins to misidentify the body's own cells as threats. This is how autoimmunity begins—not with a sudden switch, but with years of low-grade inflammation confusing the body's internal radar. Cells and tissues that should be recognized as "self" become targets, and the immune system starts to attack what it was once designed to protect. For many people, this manifests in mysterious symptoms long before a formal diagnosis is ever made: fatigue, aches, anxiety, shifting sensitivities, even depression. The effects don't stop at the immune system. Chronic inflammation can quietly sabotage your metabolism. It interferes with insulin sensitivity, makes it harder to lose weight, and increases the risk of metabolic disorders even in people who don't appear overweight. It alters how your cells take in glucose and store energy, leading to cravings, energy crashes, and that frustrating cycle of being both tired and wired. You may be eating clean and exercising, but if your body is inflamed, progress stalls. Your system is too busy fighting invisible fires to focus on healing and balance.

Your hormones, too, get pulled into the chaos. Inflammation impacts the delicate balance of estrogen, testosterone, progesterone, and thyroid hormones. It blocks hormone receptors, disrupts production pathways, and increases the conversion of beneficial hormones into more aggressive or inactive forms. For women, this might show up as irregular periods, severe PMS, or infertility. For men, it might mean low libido, weight gain, or mood changes. In both, it leads to a deep sense of disconnection from one's own vitality—and the conventional response is often to prescribe synthetic hormones rather than asking what disrupted the system in the first place.

Even your mitochondria, the tiny engines inside your cells responsible for producing energy, begin to suffer. In an inflamed state, mitochondrial function is suppressed, and the body begins to shift into an energy-conserving mode. This is why chronic inflammation is so often linked to chronic fatigue. Your body isn't just tired—it's protecting itself. It doesn't trust the current environment enough to generate full energy, because it perceives that the system is under siege.

Meanwhile, inflammation damages the endothelial lining of blood vessels, making them stickier and more prone to plaque buildup. It raises blood pressure, stiffens arteries, and contributes to the progression of cardiovascular disease. What starts as an immune response to a perceived threat eventually becomes the very process that accelerates aging. Wrinkles, cognitive decline, reduced mobility, weakened immunity—they're not just about getting older. They're the downstream effects of years spent in an inflammatory state.

What makes all this worse is that inflammation doesn't usually hurt in a way you can point to. It's insidious. You might feel off, but not ill. You might go from doctor to doctor with normal test results. You might start to believe it's all in your head. That's the great deception of inflammation: it hides in plain sight. And the longer it goes unaddressed, the more it erodes the foundation of health from the inside out.

But—and this is essential—it's not irreversible. The body is incredibly adaptive and responsive once the right signals are in place. When the inflammatory triggers are removed—when the gut is supported, the toxic burden reduced, the nervous system calmed, and the nutrients replenished—the immune system begins to shift. The fires go out. The repair mechanisms turn back on. Energy returns. Mood lifts. Symptoms fade. Health doesn't come from attacking disease; it comes from restoring the balance that inflammation disrupted in the first place.

Understanding what inflammation really does to you isn't about fear. It's about clarity. It's about finally being able to name what's been happening beneath the surface—and realizing that the answers were never out of reach. They were just hidden behind the noise.

## Why Fatigue Isn't Just 'Laziness'

Fatigue is one of the most misunderstood and dismissed symptoms in modern healthcare. It's often minimized, waved off, or reframed as a personal failing. If you're tired, the assumption is that you must not be sleeping enough, trying hard enough, moving enough, or thinking positively enough. But real fatigue—the kind that burrows deep into your bones, fogs your thoughts, and drains your drive—is not about laziness. It's a message. And it's one that the body sends when something more fundamental is out of alignment.

Chronic fatigue is not a lack of motivation. It is not weakness of character. It is not the result of poor time management or a personality flaw. It is a physiological signal that your system is in conservation mode. It's your body hitting the brakes, trying to protect what little energy it has left. And when that's ignored—or worse, pathologized as laziness—it only delays healing and deepens the exhaustion.

We live in a culture that idolizes productivity and speed. Rest is treated as a luxury or a reward, not a necessity. Many people learn early on to override the body's cues: push through the tiredness, drink more coffee, stay up late to finish work, and keep performing no matter the cost. But fatigue isn't just an inconvenience. It's an alarm system. When your cells are running low, when your brain is inflamed, when your hormones are misfiring, when your gut is out of balance—fatigue shows up to slow you down. It's one of the body's most consistent survival strategies.

There are many physiological causes behind fatigue. Mitochondrial dysfunction is one of the most overlooked. Mitochondria are the power plants of your cells. They convert nutrients into usable energy. But they are incredibly sensitive to stress, toxins, inflammation, and nutrient deficiencies. When mitochondria aren't functioning well, it doesn't matter how much you eat or sleep—your cells simply can't produce the energy you need. That's when even small tasks feel monumental. That's when you wake up tired, crash mid-morning, and can't sustain clear focus by the afternoon.

Hormonal imbalances can also contribute significantly to fatigue. When your thyroid is underactive, your metabolism slows, and fatigue becomes a constant companion. When cortisol is chronically elevated due to stress, your adrenal system becomes dysregulated—leading to a tired-but-wired feeling, poor sleep, and a slow crash over time. Women, especially, are often told that fatigue is "just part of being a woman"—tied to their cycle, their mood, or their age. But that dismissal is dangerous. Hormonal chaos is not normal, and neither is daily exhaustion.

The nervous system plays a role too. Many people today live in a state of near-constant sympathetic dominance—stuck in fight-or-flight mode. This chronic activation taxes the body's reserves. The parasympathetic state—the state of healing, digestion, and true rest—is rarely accessed. Over time, this imbalance leads to nervous system burnout. You feel tired and wired at once: restless, foggy, irritable, drained.

And yet, instead of listening to these internal signals, the system teaches us to override them. The medical establishment offers little more than vague encouragement to "get more sleep" or "exercise more," or worse, prescriptions for stimulants or antidepressants that mask symptoms without addressing root causes.

But what if fatigue isn't something to be silenced? What if it's a built-in guidance system? What if that heavy, dense feeling in your limbs isn't laziness, but the body begging for repair?

When the body signals fatigue, it's doing so with a reason. And that reason is never moral failure—it's imbalance. It's an inner ecosystem trying to recalibrate after being thrown off by toxic exposures, poor-quality sleep, inflammation, stress, blood sugar spikes, infections, emotional strain, and nutrient deficiencies. Real recovery begins when you stop fighting the fatigue and start tracing its root.

Unfortunately, many people internalize the message that being tired is unacceptable. They feel ashamed for needing to rest, for canceling plans, for not keeping up with others. That shame only compounds the problem. When fatigue becomes something to hide or power through, the body never gets the deep restoration it needs. Fatigue turns chronic.

And over time, it leads to deeper dysfunctions that are even harder to reverse.

One of the most powerful shifts you can make is to reinterpret fatigue as feedback, not failure. When you notice that your mind is foggy, your limbs heavy, your willpower depleted, that is data. It's just as valid as a fever or a swollen joint. You wouldn't blame someone with a broken leg for not running; yet we routinely blame ourselves for being tired in a broken system. And make no mistake: the system is broken.

There's a massive gap between how conventional medicine handles fatigue and what's actually required to heal from it. If your labs are "normal," you're told you're fine—even if you can't get out of bed without crashing by noon. Most standard tests don't look at mitochondrial function, inflammatory load, nutrient status, or the state of your microbiome. Fatigue is often treated like an afterthought, not a central clue.

But real practitioners, the ones who look deeper, know the pattern. They see that chronic fatigue often stems from layered dysfunctions: gut inflammation, heavy metal toxicity, stealth infections, hormone dysregulation, nervous system overload, and the emotional toll of being unheard. Healing it requires addressing all of those layers—not just trying to push harder through them.

Sleep hygiene helps, but it's rarely the full answer. Many people with chronic fatigue get enough hours in bed, yet still wake exhausted. That's because it's not just about time—it's about quality. Deep, regenerative sleep requires balance across your entire system. If cortisol is spiking at night, if your blood sugar crashes at 3 a.m., if your brain is inflamed or your liver is overburdened, your sleep will not be restful. And without true rest, your body can't repair.

Another missing piece is cellular nourishment. Fatigue often reflects a deep nutritional bankruptcy—not because people aren't eating, but because they're not absorbing. A damaged gut, constant exposure to chemicals, and stress deplete nutrients like magnesium, B vitamins, zinc, and iron. These are the building blocks your body uses to create energy.

Without them, you run on fumes, no matter how much food is on your plate.

There's also a subtle but powerful emotional layer to fatigue. When you spend years pushing through symptoms, hiding your needs, or being gaslit by the healthcare system, a quiet kind of grief settles in. It's the grief of not being believed, not being supported, not knowing why your body doesn't seem to keep up like it used to. That emotional weight is real. It's not just mental—it affects your biology. Chronic stress depletes mitochondria. Unresolved trauma disrupts hormonal rhythms. And the sheer weight of carrying unspoken exhaustion affects every system.

Healing fatigue requires validation, strategy, and time. It means honoring the signal rather than denying it. It means rebuilding your foundation— one piece at a time. Rebalancing your gut. Supporting your mitochondria. Reducing toxic exposures. Repairing your circadian rhythm. Allowing stillness without shame.

This is not about becoming "more productive." It's about becoming more attuned. When you learn to decode your body's whispers instead of silencing them, fatigue becomes less of a foe and more of a compass. It points you to what's missing, what's needed, what's next.

And that's not laziness. That's wisdom—hard-earned and finally heard.

## The Brain Fog Trap

It's a strange sensation—being present, but not fully. You're awake, but your thoughts feel sluggish, disconnected, buried under a thick mental haze. You struggle to focus, to recall the name you just heard, to finish the sentence you started. And it's not just forgetfulness. It's as if your mind is wrapped in cotton—there, but muffled. This is brain fog. And for millions of people, it's a daily, invisible struggle.

What makes brain fog so insidious is its vagueness. There's no scan that captures it, no blood marker that confirms it. You often can't explain it clearly to others, and even doctors dismiss it as stress, anxiety, or normal aging. But it's not "just in your head." It's a symptom—a real one—of deeper imbalances. And if you listen closely, brain fog is often the first sign that something in your body's operating system is under threat.

Contrary to what we've been told, clarity and mental sharpness are not privileges of youth. They're signs of internal balance. When your body is well-nourished, your gut is functioning properly, your hormones are in sync, and your immune system is calm—not overreactive—you can think clearly, process quickly, and feel mentally alive. But when one or more of those systems falls out of alignment, your brain is often the first to show it.

So many things can trigger brain fog. One of the most common—and overlooked—is blood sugar instability. Even small swings between spikes and crashes can leave your brain feeling dazed. You might eat something sugary or high-carb, get a brief mental lift, and then crash into confusion an hour later. It's not a personal weakness. It's physiology. Your brain depends on a steady stream of glucose to function. When that stream becomes erratic, your clarity disappears with it.

Then there's inflammation—particularly in the gut and brain. If your intestinal lining is compromised (what's often called "leaky gut"), toxins and food particles can slip into your bloodstream, triggering immune responses that don't stay local. They travel. And the brain—once considered a sanctuary protected by the blood-brain barrier—is now known to be vulnerable to this process. Inflammatory molecules can reach the brain and impair neurotransmission, slow processing, and dull memory. You don't feel pain in the brain like you would in your joints or muscles. You feel it as fog.

Another key player is your microbiome. Those trillions of microbes in your gut don't just help digest food—they help manufacture neurotransmitters like serotonin and dopamine, regulate immune function, and even modulate inflammation in the brain. When your microbial balance is off—due to antibiotics, processed food, chronic stress, or lack of fiber—it doesn't just affect digestion. It clouds your thinking. You might feel like your personality has changed. You become forgetful, emotionally flat, or disconnected from your own sharpness. That's not you. That's the fog.

And then there's stress. Chronic, low-grade stress reshapes the brain's chemistry. It disrupts the hypothalamic-pituitary-adrenal (HPA) axis, increasing cortisol in unpredictable waves that affect memory, sleep, and mental focus. Under stress, your brain prioritizes survival over clarity. You're not supposed to be thinking deeply when running from a lion. But in modern life, the "lion" never leaves. Notifications, deadlines, bad news, unresolved trauma—it all keeps your brain locked in reactive mode, unable to access the clarity you once had.

What traps so many people is not just the fog itself—but the shame that comes with it. You forget appointments, lose your words, reread the same sentence over and over, and quietly wonder if you're broken. Others don't see the fog. They might say you look fine. But inside, you feel slow, disconnected, not fully present. It's isolating. And it's exhausting.

You may start to question your intelligence, your work ethic, even your worth. But the truth is, brain fog is not a character flaw. It's not a sign you're lazy, disinterested, or getting old. It's a red flag from the body— a signal that something deeper needs attention. And the most powerful shift begins when you stop blaming yourself and start investigating the true causes.

Sleep, for instance, is foundational—but not just the number of hours you spend in bed. It's the *quality* of those hours. If your body isn't reaching deep, restorative sleep cycles due to stress, blood sugar instability, or hormonal imbalances, your brain doesn't get the reset it needs. You wake up groggy and spend the day chasing clarity that never comes. And no amount of coffee can replace the repair that happens during real sleep. In fact, excessive caffeine often makes the fog worse—offering a spike in energy followed by a deeper crash.

Food is another major factor. What you eat either fuels mental clarity or contributes to the fog. Processed foods, industrial seed oils, artificial additives—they may not hurt immediately, but over time, they erode the internal harmony your brain depends on. Even foods marketed as "healthy" can be inflammatory, especially when they contain hidden sugars or allergens that disrupt the gut-brain axis. Many people experience subtle cognitive shifts after eating gluten, dairy, or ultra-processed snacks without making the connection. Your brain doesn't always scream in pain—it just dims.

Hormones also play a pivotal role. Estrogen, progesterone, testosterone, insulin, thyroid hormones—they're all deeply interconnected. A shift in one can cascade across the entire system. Women, for example, often experience brain fog during perimenopause or postpartum—not because they're doing too much (though they usually are), but because their hormone levels are in flux. Men can experience similar issues with low testosterone or high cortisol. And yet, hormone testing is rarely offered unless symptoms are extreme. Fog doesn't get the same respect as disease, even though it's often the earliest whisper of one.

Many people find that when they finally begin to clean up their inputs—reducing inflammatory foods, rebalancing their microbiome, supporting liver detoxification, regulating blood sugar, and healing their sleep—the fog lifts. Not instantly, but reliably. And that's the most empowering part: this is not permanent. You're not stuck. Your clarity is not gone forever.

But getting there requires a new way of thinking. Instead of seeing the brain as separate from the body, you begin to understand that it's a mirror. If there's fog in the brain, there's almost always fire in the system—be it inflammation, imbalance, or overload. The brain is exquisitely sensitive, and its dullness is not a mystery. It's a message.

So much of modern life seems engineered to produce brain fog. Constant digital input, blue light late at night, sedentary habits, processed food, fragmented sleep—it's a perfect storm. But that also means every small shift matters. Drinking filtered water instead of sugary drinks. Moving your body daily, not for weight loss but for circulation and detox. Protecting your sleep like it's sacred. Replacing processed meals with real food. Tuning in instead of numbing out.

Clarity isn't something we're born with and slowly lose. It's something we cultivate—or forget to. And when the fog becomes chronic, it's never your fault. But it is your call to action. Because on the other side of that haze isn't just better focus. It's the return of yourself—your creativity, your memory, your spark. The ability to engage fully with life, to trust your own mind again, to feel like *you* again.

That's not too much to ask. It's the baseline you deserve. The fog was never a flaw—it was a signal. And now that you can see it, you're already on the path back to clarity.

# Part II — Breaking the Cycle

By the time most people reach their breaking point, they've already cycled through years—sometimes decades—of symptoms, confusion, frustration, and temporary fixes. They've been handed pills for pain, stimulants for energy, sedatives for sleep. Told to eat less, exercise more, "think positive," or just accept that it's aging, hormones, or stress. The result? A chronic loop. Symptoms flare, interventions suppress, deeper imbalances build, and the body becomes harder to read.

This section is about disrupting that loop—intentionally, powerfully, and without waiting for permission.

Breaking the cycle doesn't mean doing more. It means seeing clearly. It means understanding why your body has been reacting the way it has, and beginning to address the root causes that have gone ignored or misunderstood. Here, we begin to untangle the web. We look at what chronic inflammation is really doing behind the scenes—not just in joints or sinuses, but in the brain, the gut, the immune system. We examine why fatigue is *not* a personality flaw but often the result of complex internal overload. We shine a light on the signals you've been taught to brush off: the irritability after eating, the crash after coffee, the bloating, the fog, the burnout.

Every system in the body speaks its own language, but we've forgotten how to listen. Part II is where that changes. Here, we go beneath the surface. We start asking the questions most doctors don't have time—or training—to explore. What if your brain fog isn't "just stress," but a sign of blood sugar instability or microbiome disruption? What if your low energy is linked to thyroid resistance, not just low motivation? What if inflammation isn't simply a result of aging but a cascade triggered by daily exposures, toxins, or food intolerances you've never considered?

More importantly: what if it's possible to reverse it?

This part of the journey is about reclaiming your clarity, your energy, your baseline health—step by step, system by system. It's not about following another generic wellness plan. It's about understanding *why* the old patterns never worked for you, and finally learning how to work with your body instead of against it.

You'll see that the "normal" you've been living with was never truly normal—it was just common. And common is not the same as acceptable. Here, we start rewriting that narrative. We break the cycle not by pushing harder, but by getting smarter. By tuning in. By connecting the dots between your symptoms and the real internal disruptions beneath them.

And once you see it, you can't unsee it.

The cycle ends where awareness begins. This is where that begins.

# Chapter 7: Healing from Within

## Resetting Hormones Naturally

It's one of the most overlooked truths in modern health: if your hormones are out of sync, almost *everything* else will be too. Your sleep, energy, metabolism, weight, mood, libido, digestion, immunity, even your memory—they all depend on the delicate balance of chemical messengers operating behind the scenes. But thanks to chronic stress, synthetic chemicals, erratic eating patterns, and a pace of life that never lets up, this system is constantly under attack.

Resetting your hormones isn't just about "balancing estrogen" or "boosting testosterone." It's about recalibrating an entire orchestra that includes your adrenal glands, thyroid, pancreas, ovaries or testes, and your brain's regulatory centers. Each one plays a role, and when just one starts to misfire, the rest scramble to compensate. What you feel on the outside—fatigue, anxiety, weight gain, insomnia—is your body's way of alerting you that the system is no longer in harmony.

But here's the powerful truth: your body *wants* to return to balance. Hormones are not static; they respond quickly to changes in environment, behavior, and perception. This means the same system that has gone awry under stress can also recalibrate under the right conditions. And that recalibration doesn't have to involve synthetic hormones or expensive tests—it starts with restoring the natural rhythms your body was built for.

Let's begin with the master disruptor: **cortisol**, your primary stress hormone. When your brain perceives a threat—whether it's real danger, an emotional conflict, or the modern equivalent (emails, traffic, deadlines)—your adrenal glands pump out cortisol to keep you alert and ready to act. But when this signal is always on, cortisol levels remain elevated for far too long. Over time, the result is hormonal chaos: blood sugar spikes, suppressed thyroid function, disrupted ovulation, poor sleep, and constant fatigue.

What makes cortisol unique is that it doesn't just operate in the background—it *sets the tone* for every other hormone in the body. High cortisol makes your cells less responsive to insulin. It blunts the production of progesterone. It interferes with melatonin. In short, if you don't address chronic stress, no hormonal reset protocol—no matter how clean your diet or expensive your supplements—will deliver lasting results.

This is why the foundation of natural hormone reset begins with restoring **circadian rhythm** and **nervous system regulation**. Your hormonal system thrives on predictable patterns: waking and sleeping at consistent times, exposure to natural light during the day and darkness at night, eating meals at regular intervals. These may seem like minor lifestyle choices, but they are *biological levers*. Your body reads them as cues to either create balance—or perpetuate dysfunction.

One of the most overlooked factors is **blood sugar stability**. Every time your blood sugar crashes from too much caffeine, refined carbs, or skipping meals, your body sees it as a mini-emergency—and guess what hormone gets triggered? Cortisol. In turn, insulin surges to compensate, which can lead to weight gain, fatigue, and over time, insulin resistance. Keeping blood sugar steady—not too high, not too low—is one of the most efficient ways to signal to your body that it's safe, calm, and doesn't need to keep pumping stress hormones.

This interplay between food, mood, and hormones is often ignored in mainstream medicine, but it is *central* to real healing. No pill can mimic the subtle chemical signals your body creates in response to food, light, sleep, and nervous system tone. When you start tuning those levers in the right direction, the system can begin to reset itself—gently, gradually, and without forcing the body to do something unnatural.

When you consistently give your body the message that it is safe and supported—through stable blood sugar, rest, and rhythm—your hormonal system stops reacting and starts recalibrating. One of the first places this shift becomes evident is in sleep. Deep, restorative sleep isn't just a side benefit of hormone healing—it *is* hormone healing. During the night, your body releases growth hormone, repairs damaged tissues, clears inflammation, and resets cortisol levels. Without that nightly recovery cycle, you wake up depleted no matter how long you stay in bed.

Supporting natural melatonin production is essential here. That doesn't mean taking melatonin supplements every night—it means helping your body produce its own. This starts with reducing screen exposure after sunset, dimming indoor lighting, and minimizing late-night stress or stimulation. Even small adjustments like stepping outside in the morning sunlight for 10 minutes can help reset your biological clock. These may sound like lifestyle tweaks, but their effects are biochemical. Your endocrine system listens to light.

Another pillar of hormonal reset is **nourishment**—and that means more than eating "healthy." Many people unknowingly restrict the very nutrients their hormones need to function. Fats, for instance, have been demonized for decades, yet they are the raw material for sex hormones like estrogen, progesterone, and testosterone. Cholesterol, which many still fear, is the backbone of these hormones. When dietary fat is too low, or the fats consumed are highly processed (like seed oils), the body struggles to synthesize what it needs. Incorporating whole-food fats— like avocado, olive oil, pastured eggs, and wild fish—can shift this quickly.

Protein also plays a crucial role, especially for adrenal and thyroid function. Amino acids from protein-rich foods are needed to make neurotransmitters and support detoxification, two processes tightly intertwined with hormonal balance. And micronutrients like magnesium, zinc, selenium, and B vitamins act as co-factors in nearly every hormonal pathway. A deficiency in just one of these can throw off the whole cascade. When digestion is compromised—as it often is in people with chronic stress or inflammation—even the best diet may not get properly absorbed. That's why healing the gut is often a silent but necessary step in hormone repair.

Movement is another tool—not for burning calories, but for restoring hormonal communication. Overtraining or high-intensity workouts done too frequently can raise cortisol and drain the adrenals further. But gentle movement—walking, mobility work, resistance training—tells the body it's strong and adaptable without pushing it into survival mode. For many, learning to exercise *less* intensely but *more consistently* is what actually helps break the hormonal plateau.

Then there's **emotional processing**, which is rarely discussed in hormone protocols but deeply impactful. Suppressed emotions—particularly anger, grief, or chronic anxiety—can keep the body in a low-level stress state, continuously activating the hypothalamic-pituitary-adrenal (HPA) axis. This isn't about "thinking positive," but about creating space to feel, to process, to rest. Breathwork, therapy, somatic release practices—these are not extras. They are chemical interventions at the root level.

And finally, perhaps the most overlooked factor of all: **belief**. If you've been told your body is broken, that your symptoms are just age, or that nothing short of medication can help, then your nervous system may stay stuck in a defensive loop. But the body responds powerfully to permission. When you trust that it wants to heal, when you support it with the rhythms and raw materials it needs, it often responds faster than expected.

Resetting your hormones naturally isn't about chasing a single result—it's about restoring the intelligent communication network your body already possesses. It doesn't require perfection. It requires consistency, presence, and trust in the body's own timeline. And once that inner balance begins to return, the results are not only physical. There's a sense of mental clarity, emotional stability, and confidence that comes from finally feeling like your body is on your side again.

## Inflammation Recovery Through Lifestyle

We often think of inflammation as a problem to eliminate—something bad that needs suppressing. But inflammation itself isn't the enemy. It's the body's natural response to injury, stress, or perceived threat. In small doses, it's protective. The issue begins when the inflammatory response never turns off—when your body stays on high alert day after day, quietly damaging cells, organs, and systems.

The reason many people struggle to reduce chronic inflammation is because they look for a single fix—a pill, a supplement, a protocol—without realizing that healing inflammation is less about adding something new and more about removing the conditions that are keeping the fire burning. And those conditions are, more often than not, embedded in your lifestyle.

The most impactful form of recovery from chronic inflammation doesn't come from a lab. It comes from the way you live: how you eat, move, rest, and even relate to stress. This might sound simple—but it's not always easy. Because modern life is built in a way that almost guarantees low-level, persistent inflammation: processed food, poor sleep, light pollution, stress overload, toxic relationships, and sedentary habits all play a role.

Let's start with **movement**—but not the punishing, high-intensity kind. Gentle, consistent movement is one of the most powerful tools for regulating the immune system and flushing out inflammatory byproducts. When you walk, stretch, or engage in low-impact exercise, your lymphatic system gets activated. This system doesn't have a pump like your heart; it relies on muscle contractions to circulate fluid and clear waste. Without movement, toxins accumulate and inflammatory mediators stay stuck in tissues. You don't need a gym—just a body that moves daily.

Then there's **sleep**, which might be the most underrated anti-inflammatory medicine available. When your body enters deep sleep, it releases cytokines that control and downregulate inflammation. At the same time, the brain's glymphatic system clears out inflammatory debris, while cortisol levels are recalibrated to prepare for the next day. When sleep is poor or fragmented, this recovery doesn't happen. Over time, it's not just that you feel tired—your immune system becomes dysregulated, confused, and more likely to attack your own tissues.

What disrupts sleep? Blue light exposure, irregular schedules, late-night stimulation, and unresolved stress. And while many try to fix this with supplements or sleeping pills, those are short-term patches. The real solution is restoring circadian rhythm—going to bed at consistent times, reducing light exposure in the evening, allowing your body to feel safety at night. Safety, not sedation, is what creates real rest.

**Food**, of course, is a central player. But inflammation recovery through diet doesn't mean obsessively removing everything. It's not about deprivation—it's about choosing foods that speak the body's language. That means eating meals made from ingredients that the body recognizes: vegetables, fruits, healthy fats, grass-fed proteins, and fermented foods that support gut repair. It's also about reducing foods that keep the immune system triggered—ultra-processed items, seed oils, refined sugar, and chemicals that never belonged in the human diet in the first place.

But one of the least talked-about aspects of inflammation recovery is **emotional health**. The immune system doesn't live in isolation—it communicates constantly with the nervous system. When you live in a state of emotional tension, even low-grade, your brain sends signals of danger to the immune system, which then stays activated. This is why people with unresolved trauma or chronic anxiety often experience "mystery symptoms" or autoimmune flare-ups with no clear cause. Their bodies are simply responding to an emotional ecosystem that says: *you're not safe yet.*

Healing inflammation also requires a profound commitment to **stress management**, but not in the superficial way the term is often used. It's not about quick fixes or distraction techniques alone. It's about creating consistent practices that shift your nervous system out of fight-or-flight and into a state of calm safety. This is where modalities like breathwork, meditation, gentle yoga, and time in nature become more than "nice to haves"—they are essential biological tools. They teach your body that it can let down its guard, allowing immune activity to quiet and repair processes to take over.

Social connection is another powerful, yet underrated, anti-inflammatory factor. Humans evolved in communities where relationships were a cornerstone of safety and well-being. Loneliness and social isolation are now recognized as chronic stressors that activate the same inflammatory pathways as physical threats. Meaningful interactions—whether through friendships, family, or supportive groups—send signals of safety to your brain and immune system alike. Prioritizing these connections is a form of healing that nurtures both mind and body.

Environmental factors also play a significant role. The toxins we encounter daily—from polluted air to plastics and household chemicals—exert an inflammatory toll that accumulates quietly. While we can't control everything, being mindful about reducing exposure where possible—using air purifiers, choosing non-toxic products, filtering drinking water—can significantly reduce your body's inflammatory burden. Detoxification isn't about harsh cleanses; it's about lightening the load to allow your natural systems to function optimally.

One of the greatest challenges is that lifestyle changes often require consistent effort and patience, which can feel daunting when you're already exhausted or overwhelmed. But inflammation recovery isn't about perfection or overnight transformation. It's about small, sustainable shifts that compound over time. Maybe it's choosing a walk over scrolling social media. Maybe it's replacing one processed snack with a handful of nuts. Maybe it's spending five minutes outside instead of inside. These aren't trivial—they're powerful acts of self-care that whisper to your body: "You're safe. You're worth this."

Throughout this process, it's essential to practice compassion with yourself. Chronic inflammation often comes with years of wear and tear, layers of habits and exposures. Healing is rarely linear. You may have setbacks, days where symptoms flare or motivation wanes. That's not failure. It's part of the journey. Real healing honors the full human experience—both progress and pause.

Finally, inflammation recovery through lifestyle is not about replacing medical care. If you have autoimmune disease, chronic illness, or other serious conditions, working with healthcare providers remains critical. But the lifestyle foundation you build complements and enhances any treatment. It helps reduce flare-ups, improve quality of life, and may even shift the course of disease over time.

At its core, recovering from chronic inflammation through lifestyle means reclaiming agency. It means moving from feeling like a passive victim of symptoms to becoming an active participant in your healing. It's about listening deeply to your body's whispers instead of waiting for shouts. And when you commit to this path, you give yourself the best chance at not just surviving inflammation, but transcending it—returning to a state of vibrant health where your body can finally rest, repair, and thrive.

## Rebuilding Gut and Immune Resilience

Your gut is more than just a digestion machine. It's an ecosystem, a gatekeeper, and one of the central hubs of your immune system. The health of your gut and your immune resilience are intricately linked, weaving together to influence everything from your ability to fight infections to your mental clarity and energy levels. When the gut is out of balance, the immune system can become overactive, confused, or suppressed—and that's when chronic inflammation and illness start to take root.

Many modern lifestyles unknowingly damage this vital connection. Antibiotics, processed foods, stress, environmental toxins, and poor sleep erode the gut lining and disrupt the microbiome—the community of trillions of microbes living in your digestive tract. This disruption compromises the gut barrier, making it "leaky." A leaky gut allows unwanted particles like undigested food, toxins, and bacteria to pass into the bloodstream, triggering immune activation and chronic inflammation. This immune hyperactivity doesn't just affect the gut; it can cause symptoms all over the body, including fatigue, joint pain, skin issues, and brain fog.

Rebuilding gut and immune resilience requires a multifaceted approach. The first step is calming the immune system and giving your gut a chance to heal. This often means removing the triggers that keep the immune system in overdrive. Identifying and eliminating foods that irritate your gut—common culprits include gluten, dairy, soy, and processed sugars—can reduce inflammation and give the intestinal lining a chance to repair. It's not about perfection but about listening carefully to how your body reacts to different foods and choosing what supports healing. Supporting the microbiome is equally essential. A diverse and balanced gut flora trains your immune system to respond appropriately. Fermented foods like sauerkraut, kimchi, kefir, and yogurt introduce beneficial bacteria, while prebiotic fibers from vegetables, legumes, and whole grains feed those microbes. Avoiding unnecessary antibiotics and minimizing exposure to antibacterial products also helps preserve this delicate ecosystem.

Beyond diet, stress management is a critical factor. The gut and brain communicate through the vagus nerve, forming the gut-brain axis. Chronic stress disrupts this communication, increasing gut permeability and altering microbiome composition. Mind-body practices such as meditation, gentle yoga, and breathwork have been shown to support gut healing by reducing stress hormones and improving vagal tone.

Nutrients play a foundational role as well. Healing the gut lining requires amino acids like glutamine, which helps repair epithelial cells. Minerals such as zinc and selenium support immune regulation, while omega-3 fatty acids reduce inflammation. Vitamin D, often deficient in modern populations, is a powerful modulator of immune function and gut health. Ensuring adequate intake of these nutrients through food or supplementation can accelerate recovery.

In some cases, targeted probiotics can help restore balance, but they should be chosen carefully and ideally under guidance. Not all probiotics are created equal, and introducing the wrong strains can sometimes worsen symptoms. Healing the gut is a journey of trial and observation, paying attention to what your body needs.

Finally, patience is key. The gut lining takes time to rebuild—often weeks to months—and immune retraining is a gradual process. You may notice improvements in digestion and energy first, while other symptoms like skin or joint issues take longer to resolve. The body is complex, and healing unfolds in layers. It requires consistent care and kindness.

As you continue to nurture your gut and support immune balance, other factors come into play that often go unnoticed but can make a significant difference. Sleep quality, for instance, deeply affects gut health and immune function. During restorative sleep, the body repairs the intestinal lining, recalibrates immune responses, and reduces inflammation. Without adequate sleep, these processes falter, leaving your gut vulnerable and your immune system primed for overreaction.

Hydration is another key component. Water supports digestion, flushes toxins, and maintains the mucosal lining of the intestines. Drinking clean, filtered water helps keep the gut environment balanced and supports the efficient removal of metabolic waste that can trigger immune responses.

Physical activity, when balanced correctly, acts as a natural anti-inflammatory. Movement increases blood flow and lymphatic drainage, which aids in removing toxins and reducing immune activation. However, overexertion or excessive high-intensity exercise can stress the body and worsen inflammation. Gentle, consistent movement like walking, stretching, or yoga is often the best approach during gut healing. Environmental exposures also influence immune resilience. Household chemicals, air pollution, and plastics carry compounds that disrupt gut bacteria and challenge immune tolerance. Minimizing contact with these toxins by using natural cleaning products, improving indoor air quality, and reducing plastic use can alleviate this hidden stress on your system.

Emotional health remains a powerful driver in gut and immune recovery. Chronic anxiety or unresolved trauma creates a persistent state of alertness, releasing stress hormones that increase intestinal permeability and promote inflammation. Engaging in therapies that address emotional wounds—such as somatic therapy, mindfulness, or talk therapy—can facilitate healing on this unseen but vital front.

As your gut lining strengthens and microbiome diversity increases, you'll likely notice shifts in your symptoms. Digestive discomfort may ease, skin conditions may improve, and energy levels can stabilize. Mental clarity often returns as gut-brain communication normalizes, helping to clear brain fog and reduce anxiety or depression linked to inflammation. At this stage, some find it helpful to integrate targeted supplements designed to support gut repair and immune modulation. Components like collagen peptides provide building blocks for the intestinal lining, while compounds such as L-glutamine nourish the cells that form your gut barrier. Herbal anti-inflammatories—like turmeric and ginger—can further soothe immune activation. Probiotics tailored to your unique microbiome profile may assist in restoring balance, but these should complement, not replace, foundational lifestyle changes.

Remember, healing the gut and rebuilding immune resilience is a marathon, not a sprint. It requires patience, consistency, and attention to subtle feedback from your body. Some days will feel like progress; others may feel like setbacks. This ebb and flow is natural and reflects the complexity of the systems involved.

Above all, reclaiming your gut and immune health is an act of self-trust and empowerment. It means learning to listen deeply to your body's signals and responding with compassion rather than judgment. The journey may challenge old beliefs about health and productivity, but the reward is profound: a body that functions with resilience, a mind that feels clear, and an immune system that supports rather than sabotages your well-being.

This renewed foundation doesn't just reduce symptoms—it creates the conditions for vibrant health to flourish. Your gut and immune system are your allies, not your enemies. When you care for them with intention, you open the door to lasting vitality, balance, and freedom from chronic inflammation.

# Chapter 8: Food as a Foundation

## Whole Foods vs. Frankenstein Foods

In a world saturated with packaged products, convenience meals, and industrially processed snacks, the battle between whole foods and what might be called "Frankenstein foods" has never been more relevant. But what do these terms really mean? And why does this distinction matter so profoundly for your health, energy, and even longevity?

Whole foods are foods in their most natural, unaltered state—fresh vegetables, fruits, nuts, seeds, whole grains, legumes, and properly sourced meats and fish. They are complex, living packages of nutrition, rich in fiber, vitamins, minerals, antioxidants, and beneficial phytochemicals. Each bite offers a symphony of nutrients that your body recognizes, digests, and uses to sustain cellular function and systemic balance.

Frankenstein foods, on the other hand, are the products of industrial food engineering. They are often stripped of natural components—fiber, micronutrients, and enzymes—and then reassembled with artificial additives, preservatives, emulsifiers, flavor enhancers, and refined ingredients. These products are designed for shelf stability, low cost, and hyper-palatability, not for nourishment.

The rise of Frankenstein foods has paralleled the explosion of chronic health issues—obesity, diabetes, autoimmune disease, mental health struggles, and digestive disorders. While it's tempting to attribute these epidemics to "lifestyle" in a general sense, the quality of what we eat sits at the center. When your diet is dominated by highly processed, synthetic-laden foods, your body doesn't just lack nutrients—it is actively burdened by substances it can't recognize or safely eliminate.

One of the fundamental problems with Frankenstein foods is their impact on the gut microbiome. The bacteria and other microbes living in your digestive tract thrive on diversity and fiber-rich foods. Whole plant foods provide an array of fermentable fibers and polyphenols that feed beneficial bacteria, encouraging a balanced microbiome. Processed foods, however, are often stripped of fiber and packed with sugar, unhealthy fats, and chemical additives that disrupt microbial balance, promote inflammation, and compromise gut integrity.

The damage extends beyond the gut. Frankenfoods typically contain industrial seed oils—like soybean, corn, and canola oils—that are high in omega-6 fatty acids. While omega-6 fats are essential in small amounts, an imbalance skewed heavily toward omega-6 can fuel chronic inflammation. These oils are highly unstable, prone to oxidation and free radical formation during processing and cooking, further increasing oxidative stress in the body.

Sugar, another hallmark of processed foods, spikes blood glucose and insulin repeatedly throughout the day, which not only creates energy crashes but also promotes systemic inflammation and insulin resistance. The body's delicate hormonal balance is challenged constantly, and the brain suffers from erratic fuel supply—both of which contribute to fatigue, fog, and metabolic chaos.

Perhaps most concerning is the presence of synthetic additives—flavor enhancers, artificial colors, preservatives, and emulsifiers—that have been shown in emerging research to alter gut permeability, disrupt hormonal signaling, and provoke immune reactions. These ingredients are foreign to human biology and can confuse the body's complex regulatory systems, leading to what many experience as "unexplained" symptoms: digestive upset, brain fog, skin rashes, and mood swings.

The paradox of modern food is that while we have never had more access to calories, we have never been more nutrient deficient. Calories are easy to come by in processed foods, but real nutrition is scarce. Whole foods, by contrast, offer a dense package of nutrition that supports every cell, organ, and system. They provide the raw materials your body needs to detoxify, repair, and thrive. They promote satiety and steady blood sugar, which helps regulate mood and energy.

The solution, however, isn't simply about "cutting out junk" or following the latest fad diet. It's about reconnecting with food as a source of healing and vitality. It's about choosing foods that nourish your unique body and honor your natural rhythms. It's about understanding the impact of food choices on your microbiome, immune system, and hormonal health.

Many people feel overwhelmed by the thought of making such changes. Convenience, taste preferences, social pressures, and misinformation all create barriers. But the transition doesn't have to be all or nothing. Small shifts—like swapping out refined snacks for nuts, adding an extra serving of vegetables, cooking more meals at home—accumulate and create lasting change.

The shift toward whole foods isn't just a trend—it's a return to biology. When you choose whole, minimally processed foods, you're feeding not only yourself but also the trillions of microbes that inhabit your gut. This symbiotic relationship affects digestion, immune response, inflammation, and even mental health. Beneficial bacteria break down fibers into short-chain fatty acids that nourish the gut lining and regulate immune tolerance. This harmony is disrupted when processed foods dominate, leading to imbalance and vulnerability.

The impact of Frankenfoods extends beyond nutrition. The way these products are engineered tricks your brain's reward system. Ultra-processed foods are designed to be hyper-palatable—they combine fat, sugar, salt, and artificial flavor enhancers in ways that overstimulate dopamine pathways. This creates cravings and overeating, reinforcing patterns that keep you tied to the very foods that undermine your health. It's a cycle that's hard to break without awareness.

Moreover, industrial farming and food manufacturing practices contribute to nutrient depletion. Soil depletion means even "whole" foods can be less nutrient-dense than in previous generations. Add to that the widespread use of pesticides and herbicides, which may further disturb gut microbiota and immune function, and the challenge becomes clearer: we have to be intentional not only about *what* we eat but *how* it is grown and sourced.

Cooking methods matter as well. High-heat frying, microwaving, and prolonged storage can oxidize fats and degrade nutrients, turning even some whole foods into inflammatory triggers. Embracing gentle cooking methods—steaming, roasting, slow simmering—and eating some foods raw preserves their nutritional integrity and supports your body's healing processes.

Transitioning to a whole foods-based diet can feel overwhelming in today's fast-paced culture. But it's worth remembering that your choices are also acts of self-care and resistance against a system that prioritizes profit over health. Simple practices, like meal prepping, prioritizing seasonal produce, and exploring traditional food preparation methods, can create a sustainable, nourishing routine.

Finally, whole foods bring a sense of connection. Cooking and eating whole foods invite you into a relationship with your body and the environment. They encourage mindfulness, gratitude, and respect for the life cycle that sustains us. This deeper connection fosters not only physical health but also emotional and spiritual well-being—elements often missing in modern health narratives.

Choosing whole foods over Frankenstein foods isn't about perfection or restriction—it's about reclaiming your health from the ground up. It's about nourishing your cells, calming your immune system, supporting your hormones, and reclaiming your mental clarity. It's a profound act of alignment with the biology that has evolved over millennia—an invitation to thrive rather than merely survive.

The foods you choose are among your most powerful allies on this journey. When you honor them, your body responds with vitality, resilience, and balance. And that is the foundation for everything else that follows.

## What to Remove and What to Rebuild

One of the biggest challenges in reclaiming your health is knowing where to begin. Chronic symptoms often come tangled in layers of lifestyle, environment, and biology. It's easy to feel overwhelmed by the sheer number of factors that could be contributing to your fatigue, brain fog, or inflammation. But the key to lasting transformation lies in two foundational steps: removing what harms and rebuilding what supports. The first step is about **removal**—identifying and reducing the sources of ongoing stress and toxicity that keep your body locked in imbalance. This is not about drastic detoxes or extreme restriction. It's about mindful, practical actions that decrease the burden on your system so it can begin to heal.

One of the most important targets for removal is **dietary triggers**. Foods that inflame the gut, disrupt blood sugar, or burden detox pathways need to be reduced or eliminated temporarily. Common culprits include refined sugars, processed seed oils, gluten, dairy, and artificial additives. These foods may not cause obvious immediate reactions but can sustain low-grade inflammation and immune activation over time. Removing them gives your gut lining a chance to repair and your immune system a chance to calm.

Environmental toxins also demand attention. Chemicals in household cleaners, personal care products, plastics, and air pollution accumulate silently in your body. While it's impossible to avoid all exposures, you can reduce your load by choosing natural or non-toxic alternatives, improving indoor air quality, and filtering your water. Every small reduction in toxin exposure lessens the stress on your liver and immune system.

Another layer to remove is **chronic stress**. This isn't just about big life events—it's the daily grind, the constant noise of digital devices, emotional tension, and unresolved trauma that keep your nervous system on high alert. Managing this kind of stress requires practices that cultivate safety and rest, like meditation, breathwork, and boundary-setting. It's a gradual process but essential for stopping the continuous cortisol flood that sabotages your hormonal and immune balance.

Sleep disruption is another factor to address. Even subtle irregularities in sleep-wake cycles can maintain inflammation and impair recovery. Removing habits that interfere with restful sleep—late-night screen time, irregular bedtimes, caffeine after noon—creates space for your body's natural repair rhythms.

Once harmful influences are reduced, the next step is **rebuilding**— supporting the systems that maintain health and resilience. This means nourishing your body with what it needs to restore balance.

Nutrient-dense whole foods form the cornerstone of rebuilding. These provide the vitamins, minerals, and antioxidants your cells require to detoxify, repair DNA, balance hormones, and calm inflammation. Focus on fresh vegetables, healthy fats, quality proteins, and fermented foods to support gut health and immune function.

Supporting your **gut microbiome** is critical. A diverse and thriving community of beneficial bacteria trains your immune system, produces vital nutrients, and protects the gut lining. Rebuilding this community means feeding it with prebiotic fibers—found in asparagus, garlic, onions, and resistant starches—and introducing beneficial microbes through fermented foods and targeted probiotics when appropriate.

Restoration also involves supporting your **liver and detox pathways**. The liver is your body's primary filter for environmental toxins and metabolic waste. Nutrients like glutathione precursors, B vitamins, and sulfur-containing foods (like cruciferous vegetables) enhance its function. Gentle movement and sweating through exercise or sauna use also aid detoxification.

Rebuilding your **nervous system** requires intentional restoration of the parasympathetic (rest-and-digest) state. Regular practices that promote relaxation and presence—mindful breathing, yoga, meditation, time in nature—help regulate the HPA axis, reduce cortisol, and calm immune overactivation.

Finally, rebuilding is about cultivating **consistency and compassion**. Healing is rarely a straight line. You will have good days and setbacks.

Recognizing this with kindness rather than frustration fosters resilience and keeps you engaged in the process.

Rebuilding also means restoring your relationship with your body and your environment. So often, chronic symptoms create a sense of disconnection—from our own physical sensations, from nature, and even from our community. This estrangement itself becomes a source of stress, perpetuating inflammation and hormonal imbalance. Taking intentional time to reconnect—to move mindfully, breathe deeply, and simply be present—signals to your nervous system that you are safe. It rewires stress pathways and opens space for healing.

Another powerful aspect of rebuilding is nurturing **emotional resilience**. Chronic stress and trauma don't just impact the mind; they embed themselves in the body's physiology, affecting immune function and hormonal regulation. Practices that support emotional processing—such as journaling, therapy, or somatic work—can release stored tension and help you reclaim a sense of control over your health journey. Healing isn't only about what you add or remove externally but also about how you relate internally.

It's important to recognize that removal and rebuilding are ongoing processes, not one-time actions. New stressors will inevitably arise, old habits may creep back in, and life's unpredictability will test your progress. But with a strong foundation rooted in awareness and intention, you'll be equipped to respond rather than react—to course-correct rather than collapse.

The integration of these strategies creates a **feedback loop**: as you remove harmful inputs, your body feels less burdened; as you rebuild supportive systems, your resilience increases; and as resilience grows, your capacity to tolerate and adapt to life's challenges strengthens. This loop isn't just physical—it touches every part of your experience, from your energy levels and mood to your relationships and sense of purpose.

You don't have to tackle everything at once. In fact, trying to do so often leads to overwhelm and burnout. Instead, choose one or two areas to focus on at a time. Maybe it's starting with sleep hygiene and reducing processed foods. Maybe it's committing to gentle daily movement or creating a calming bedtime ritual. These small, sustainable changes ripple outwards, building momentum that carries you forward.

Support systems—whether professional, social, or community-based—also play a critical role in rebuilding. Working with practitioners who understand the complexities of chronic symptoms can provide guidance, validation, and accountability. Connecting with others on similar journeys reminds you that you are not alone, reducing isolation and inspiring hope.

Finally, embrace patience. The body's systems have often been under strain for months or years before symptoms emerge. Healing takes time. But that time is well spent. Each step you take towards removing what harms and rebuilding what supports is a step towards freedom from chronic illness and a return to vibrant life.

Remember, you are not broken. You are responding to conditions that need changing. And with intention, awareness, and compassion, you can rewrite your body's story—transforming challenge into opportunity and exhaustion into vitality.

# The Truth About Supplements

In the quest for better health, supplements often feel like the easy answer. When symptoms pile up and energy flags, the promise of a pill that can restore balance or plug nutritional gaps is tempting. The supplement industry, worth billions, is built on this appeal—marketing "miracle" vitamins, minerals, herbs, and formulas that claim to fix everything from fatigue to brain fog to hormonal imbalance.

But the truth about supplements is far more nuanced. They are tools—sometimes powerful, sometimes unnecessary, sometimes even harmful—depending on how they're used. Supplements are not magic bullets. They don't replace a healthy diet or lifestyle. And they certainly don't work the same for everyone.

One of the biggest misconceptions is that taking more supplements automatically equals better health. In reality, your body has a remarkable ability to absorb and utilize nutrients from whole foods, where vitamins and minerals come paired with co-factors, fiber, and other compounds that enhance bioavailability. When you isolate nutrients in a pill, you often lose that synergy. In some cases, supplements can compete for absorption, interfere with medications, or lead to imbalances if taken in excess.

Another important point is that supplements should be tailored, not generic. The human body is complex and unique. Nutrient needs vary widely depending on age, genetics, health status, lifestyle, and underlying imbalances. What helps one person might do nothing—or even cause harm—for another. That's why indiscriminate use of multivitamins or "superfood" blends can be ineffective or counterproductive.

Testing plays a critical role in responsible supplementation. Blood work, functional assessments, and careful symptom tracking help identify specific deficiencies or imbalances that need addressing. For example, low vitamin D or magnesium levels are common and often benefit from targeted supplementation. But taking high doses of these nutrients without guidance can create new problems or mask symptoms without resolving the underlying causes.

It's also essential to understand the quality of supplements. Not all brands are created equal. Some products contain fillers, binders, or contaminants. Others use synthetic forms of nutrients that the body doesn't absorb well. Choosing reputable brands that prioritize transparency, third-party testing, and high-quality ingredients makes a significant difference.

Supplements are best viewed as a bridge—a way to support the body while foundational lifestyle factors are addressed. They can accelerate healing when used judiciously but are rarely sufficient on their own. For example, someone with chronic fatigue and poor gut health might benefit from a probiotic or digestive enzymes, but without improving diet, sleep, and stress, supplements alone won't restore vitality.

Many herbal supplements also deserve a careful approach. While plants have been used medicinally for centuries, modern extraction methods and dosing vary widely. Herbs like adaptogens (ashwagandha, rhodiola), anti-inflammatories (turmeric, ginger), and nervines (chamomile, valerian) can support hormonal balance and nervous system resilience, but only when integrated thoughtfully into a broader health plan.

Overreliance on supplements can sometimes create a false sense of security, leading people to neglect crucial lifestyle changes. This mindset can stall progress, resulting in frustration when symptoms persist despite a cabinet full of pills. True healing requires a shift from a "quick fix" mentality to a deeper commitment to listening to and supporting your body's needs holistically.

Finally, supplements can sometimes interact with medications or other supplements, creating unexpected effects. That's why consulting healthcare professionals—especially those experienced in integrative or functional medicine—is critical before starting any new supplement regimen.

It's important to approach supplements with a mindset of respect and curiosity rather than expectation. They can provide targeted support during times when your body is under stress, recovering from illness, or dealing with specific deficiencies. For example, supplementing with vitamin B12 can be life-changing for those with absorption issues, while omega-3 fatty acids support brain health and reduce inflammation. But even the best supplements aren't meant to be a substitute for nourishing whole foods, quality sleep, regular movement, or stress management.

Education plays a critical role in navigating the vast supplement market. The language can be confusing—terms like "bioavailability," "standardized extracts," "isomers," and "fillers" are often overlooked but carry great significance for effectiveness and safety. Learning to read labels critically, understanding what each ingredient does, and knowing which forms are most usable by the body empowers you to make informed choices that align with your health goals.

Supplement timing and dosage are also crucial. Taking supplements sporadically or in improper amounts can limit their benefits or cause side effects. For instance, fat-soluble vitamins like A, D, E, and K require dietary fat for absorption, so taking them on an empty stomach or with low-fat meals diminishes their impact. Similarly, some supplements, such as magnesium, have a calming effect and are best taken in the evening, while others, like B vitamins, may be more energizing and better suited for morning use.

Personal experimentation, guided by professional advice and self-awareness, helps identify which supplements support your unique biology. Tracking how you feel after starting or stopping a supplement can provide valuable insights. Sometimes, what works during one phase of life or health condition may need adjusting later. Your body's needs are dynamic, and supplement protocols should evolve accordingly.

A balanced approach also includes knowing when to stop. Prolonged use of certain supplements without reassessment can lead to imbalances or dependency. For example, excessive zinc supplementation can interfere with copper absorption, and high doses of antioxidants might blunt necessary oxidative processes involved in cellular repair. Periodic breaks and cycles of supplementation, combined with retesting when appropriate, ensure you're supporting your body's rhythms rather than overriding them.

Another truth is that supplements are just one piece of a larger puzzle. Many health challenges stem from systemic issues that require comprehensive lifestyle shifts. Detoxifying environmental exposures, improving sleep hygiene, rebuilding gut health, managing emotional stress, and eating nutrient-dense whole foods often provide more profound and lasting improvements than any supplement can deliver alone.

Finally, cultivating patience and realistic expectations is vital. Supplements can aid recovery and optimize function, but they don't produce overnight miracles. The body's healing is a gradual process—sometimes subtle, sometimes dramatic—but always unique. Giving your body the time and consistent care it needs, while using supplements judiciously, creates the foundation for sustainable health.

Supplements can be allies on your journey, but only when used thoughtfully, individually, and as part of a holistic plan. They're tools to empower you, not magic bullets to bypass the deeper work. When you understand their role and respect their limits, you harness their true potential—supporting your body gently, effectively, and safely toward vibrant wellness.

# Chapter 9: Movement, Sleep, and Reconnection

## Why Movement Matters More Than Exercise

When most people think about physical activity, their minds jump to exercise—the gym, intense workouts, running, or classes designed to push your limits. But there's a vital distinction that often goes unspoken: movement and exercise are not the same. Movement is the simple, natural action of using your body in varied ways throughout the day. Exercise is structured, goal-oriented, and often intense. And while exercise can be beneficial, movement—consistent, varied, and gentle— plays a far greater role in long-term health and healing.

Our bodies evolved for movement in natural environments: walking, climbing, reaching, bending, carrying, balancing. This kind of movement is low intensity but frequent, varied in pattern, and integral to daily living. Modern life, with its hours spent sitting, repetitive motions, and limited physical variety, robs us of this essential movement. This deprivation doesn't just weaken muscles—it disrupts circulation, lymph flow, nervous system regulation, and even cellular repair processes.

Movement matters because it's how your body communicates health to every system within it. When you move regularly throughout the day, you stimulate blood flow that delivers oxygen and nutrients to cells and carries away toxins. You activate your lymphatic system, which helps clear waste and regulate immune responses. You engage your nervous system in ways that signal safety and vitality, reducing stress hormones and supporting hormonal balance. These benefits don't require a gym membership or an intense sweat session—they happen with simple, consistent motion.

The problem is that many people wait until they "have time for exercise" or feel motivated to "work out." But that's not how movement works. Your body thrives on variety and consistency. Sitting for long stretches, even if you do a 45-minute workout once a day, leaves you deprived of

106

the movement your cells crave. This is why "sitting disease" is now recognized as a major health risk—because sedentary behavior undermines the very systems that exercise only partially supports.

Another crucial factor is that excessive or inappropriate exercise can sometimes do more harm than good. High-intensity workouts, especially if done without adequate recovery, raise cortisol levels, increase inflammation, and stress the nervous system. For those struggling with chronic fatigue, inflammation, or hormonal imbalance, pushing hard can perpetuate the very cycles they're trying to break. Movement, on the other hand, is gentle enough to support healing yet powerful enough to stimulate positive changes in circulation, metabolism, and mood.

The type of movement also matters. Activities that promote **functional movement**—like walking barefoot on natural surfaces, stretching, gentle yoga, balance exercises, and light strength training—encourage mobility, flexibility, and nervous system regulation. These varied movements counteract the repetitive, unnatural patterns that modern life imposes on the body. They help reset posture, improve joint health, and enhance proprioception (your body's ability to sense position and movement), all of which reduce injury risk and improve quality of life.

For many, the goal isn't to become an athlete but to reclaim basic physical freedom and resilience. Simple habits like standing up and walking every hour, taking the stairs instead of the elevator, playing with pets or children, gardening, or stretching at your desk add meaningful movement that accumulates into significant health benefits. These acts also create opportunities for mindfulness, grounding, and stress relief, further amplifying their healing power.

Importantly, movement fosters a positive feedback loop with mental health. Physical activity, even mild, triggers the release of endorphins and neurotransmitters like serotonin and dopamine, which elevate mood and reduce anxiety. Unlike the pressure some feel around "working out," movement can be joyful, playful, and nurturing. It reconnects you with your body in a way that builds confidence and presence, rather than stress or obligation.

Recognizing the difference between movement and exercise also opens the door to redefining success in physical activity. Success isn't measured solely by the number of calories burned or the intensity of a workout but by how well your body functions in daily life and how you feel overall. Can you move with ease? Do your joints feel supple and your muscles balanced? Are you able to engage your nervous system in a way that fosters calm and vitality? These are the true markers of physical health.

This perspective shifts the focus from rare, intense exertion to consistent, enjoyable movement integrated naturally into your routine. Consider activities like walking outdoors, gentle stretching, or even dancing around your kitchen—these don't just burn calories; they nurture circulation, support lymphatic drainage, improve mood, and activate the parasympathetic nervous system. Over time, these movements build resilience without triggering stress responses.

For those dealing with chronic fatigue, inflammation, or hormonal imbalances, prioritizing movement over intense exercise can be transformative. It respects your current energy limits while encouraging progression. Movement becomes a form of listening—honoring what your body can do today and gently expanding its capacity. This sustainable approach prevents burnout and fosters long-term adherence.

Another often-overlooked benefit of movement is its role in **gut health**. Physical activity promotes healthy digestion and motility, reducing bloating and supporting a balanced microbiome. Unlike high-intensity exercise that can sometimes stress the gut, moderate movement encourages parasympathetic activation, aiding in nutrient absorption and waste elimination—both vital for recovery from chronic inflammation.

Moreover, movement enhances **brain health** through increased blood flow, oxygenation, and the release of neurotrophic factors that support cognitive function. This isn't just about physical benefits; it's about reclaiming mental clarity and emotional stability. Gentle, varied movement helps reduce brain fog and anxiety, creating a positive cycle that supports the holistic healing process.

Incorporating movement also builds a deeper connection to your body, fostering mindfulness and presence. This embodied awareness is crucial for noticing subtle shifts, responding to early signs of imbalance, and cultivating compassion for yourself through the healing journey. Movement becomes a dialogue rather than a prescription—a way to co-create health rather than chase unattainable ideals.

Practical steps to increase movement don't require special equipment or memberships. Simple changes like standing or walking during phone calls, taking short breaks to stretch, gardening, or playing with pets contribute meaningful activity. Embracing movement as a daily practice rather than an occasional event ensures that your body remains engaged and vibrant.

It's also important to acknowledge cultural and social barriers that can make movement challenging for many. Time constraints, access to safe spaces, and past experiences with exercise can create resistance or discomfort. Recognizing these obstacles without judgment and seeking enjoyable, personalized ways to move fosters sustainability and joy.

Ultimately, valuing movement over exercise is about aligning with your body's natural design and rhythms. It's a call to move with intention, kindness, and curiosity—choosing activities that honor where you are right now while gently inviting growth. This approach dismantles the "all or nothing" mindset and replaces it with a balanced, nourishing relationship to your physical self.

When movement is integrated thoughtfully, it becomes a powerful pillar of healing—supporting circulation, reducing inflammation, regulating hormones, and restoring nervous system balance. It sets the stage for improved sleep, enhanced energy, and greater resilience against life's stressors.

The journey toward health is rarely linear, but embracing movement as a daily, joyful practice creates momentum that carries you forward. This simple shift—prioritizing consistent, varied movement over sporadic intense exercise—can transform how you feel, think, and live.

And that transformation is the foundation of vibrant, lasting wellness.

## The Real Role of Sleep in Healing

Sleep is often underestimated in conversations about health and healing, treated as a passive state or a simple nightly pause. But sleep is far from idle. It is a dynamic, vital process during which your body performs some of its most critical restoration and maintenance functions. Understanding the real role of sleep reveals why it is foundational to recovering from chronic fatigue, inflammation, hormonal imbalance, and brain fog.

The body's systems do not shut down when you sleep. Instead, they shift into repair mode. Your immune system ramps up the production of infection-fighting cells and molecules. Inflammation is reduced as pro-inflammatory cytokines drop and anti-inflammatory agents increase. Damage from daily oxidative stress begins to heal. At the same time, your brain's glymphatic system activates to flush out neurotoxins and metabolic waste that accumulate during waking hours. This clearing process is essential for maintaining cognitive function and preventing neurodegenerative diseases.

Hormonal regulation is tightly linked to sleep quality and quantity. During deep sleep stages, the pituitary gland releases growth hormone, which supports tissue repair, muscle growth, and metabolism. Melatonin, the sleep hormone, not only regulates circadian rhythms but also functions as a powerful antioxidant. Cortisol, the primary stress hormone, naturally dips at night, allowing the body to rest. Disrupted or insufficient sleep interferes with these rhythms, causing a cascade of hormonal imbalances that affect energy, mood, and immune responses.

Sleep cycles through different stages—light sleep, deep restorative sleep, and REM sleep, which is crucial for emotional processing and memory consolidation. The balance and length of these cycles determine how refreshed and healed you feel upon waking. Fragmented sleep or insufficient time spent in these key stages leads to symptoms like brain fog, irritability, and fatigue, which are often mistaken for other issues.

Modern lifestyle factors disrupt this intricate dance. Artificial light exposure, especially blue light from screens, suppresses melatonin production and delays sleep onset. Irregular sleep schedules confuse the body's internal clock, leading to poor alignment with natural circadian rhythms. Stress and anxiety keep the nervous system in a heightened state, making it difficult to transition into restful sleep. Even diet and exercise timing can affect how well you sleep.

The consequences of chronic sleep disruption go beyond feeling tired. Sleep deprivation impairs glucose metabolism and increases insulin resistance, contributing to weight gain and diabetes risk. It elevates inflammatory markers, aggravating autoimmune and chronic inflammatory conditions. Memory, creativity, and emotional resilience suffer. Over time, poor sleep accelerates aging processes and increases vulnerability to disease.

Despite this, many people rely on caffeine, energy drinks, or stimulants to "power through" their days, perpetuating a vicious cycle of exhaustion and poor rest. Others turn to sleeping pills, which may offer short-term relief but often do not restore natural sleep architecture or support long-term healing. The key to leveraging sleep for recovery lies in creating conditions that allow your body's innate systems to function optimally.

Establishing a **consistent sleep routine** aligned with natural light-dark cycles is foundational. Going to bed and waking up at the same time daily supports circadian regulation. Creating a sleep-friendly environment—cool, dark, and quiet—further signals safety to the brain. Reducing screen time and artificial lighting at least an hour before bed helps restore melatonin production.

Addressing stress through mindfulness practices, breathwork, or gentle movement calms the nervous system, making it easier to fall and stay asleep. Avoiding heavy meals, caffeine, and intense exercise close to bedtime prevents sleep disturbances. In some cases, supplements like magnesium or herbal nervines can assist, but these should complement—not replace—behavioral strategies.

The real role of sleep in healing is not just about quantity but quality, consistency, and alignment with your body's natural rhythms. When you honor sleep as a critical pillar of health, you unlock your body's potential to repair, detoxify, and restore balance—laying the groundwork for vibrant energy, clear thinking, and emotional well-being.

While the mechanics of sleep are complex, the path to better rest often begins with reclaiming a sense of safety and rhythm in your life. Modern stressors—constant notifications, overwhelming to-do lists, and the pressure to be "always on"—keep your nervous system in a state of hypervigilance. This state is the antithesis of restorative sleep. Training your nervous system to relax requires more than just "trying to fall asleep." It demands intentional practices that help you unwind physically, mentally, and emotionally before bedtime.

Creating a calming pre-sleep routine can be transformative. Activities like gentle stretching, reading printed books, practicing mindful breathing, or soaking in a warm bath signal to your brain that it's time to shift gears. These rituals replace the chaos of the day with a sequence of predictable, soothing actions that prepare your body for repair.

Nutrition also influences sleep quality. Eating a balanced diet that stabilizes blood sugar throughout the day helps prevent nighttime awakenings. Heavy meals or sugar spikes late in the evening can disrupt your sleep cycles and trigger cortisol release. Certain nutrients—magnesium, B vitamins, and tryptophan-rich foods—support neurotransmitter production essential for sleep regulation. Incorporating these can gently support your body's natural rhythms.

Addressing underlying health conditions is equally important. Chronic pain, digestive issues, hormonal imbalances, and mental health challenges can all interfere with sleep. Instead of viewing poor sleep as a standalone problem, recognizing it as a symptom invites a more comprehensive approach. Treating the root causes enhances sleep, which in turn accelerates healing across systems.

It's crucial to move away from quick fixes like sedatives or excessive caffeine, which often mask deeper issues and degrade sleep quality over time. Instead, focus on lifestyle and environmental factors that empower your body to self-regulate. This approach fosters not only better sleep but a renewed capacity for resilience during waking hours.

Tracking sleep patterns—through journals or wearable devices—can provide valuable insights. Noticing trends around what helps or hinders your rest allows for targeted adjustments. Remember, improvement can be gradual. Patience with your body's unique pace is an essential part of the process.

Ultimately, the real role of sleep in healing goes far beyond rest. It is a master regulator of health, influencing immune function, hormonal balance, detoxification, and brain clarity. Prioritizing sleep as a foundational pillar—equally important as nutrition, movement, and stress management—unlocks the potential for deep, lasting transformation.

When you honor sleep's true purpose and nurture the conditions it needs, you create a powerful environment for your body to heal from the inside out. This is not indulgence; it is essential care. In this space, your body rebuilds, your mind clears, and your spirit renews—preparing you to meet each day with restored energy and clarity.

## Reconnecting to the Body's Signals

In the whirlwind of modern life, many people have lost touch with one of their most vital resources: their own body's signals. Fatigue, pain, hunger, stress—these sensations are meant to be guides, messages from the body alerting us to needs, imbalances, or boundaries. But when we ignore, suppress, or misinterpret these signals, we disconnect from an essential feedback loop, making healing far more difficult.

The disconnect often begins early. Cultural norms encourage pushing through discomfort, dismissing tiredness as laziness, or "powering through" stress without pause. Over time, this rewires the nervous system to tolerate higher levels of stress and discomfort as normal, blunting sensitivity to subtle signals. What starts as a whisper—a slight headache, a twinge of pain, a vague sense of unease—becomes drowned out by the noise of daily demands.

Reconnecting to your body's signals requires patience and intention. It's a process of relearning how to listen without judgment or fear. The goal is not to become hyper-aware or anxious about every sensation, but to cultivate a gentle curiosity—a respectful attention to what your body tells you and a willingness to respond with care.

One of the first steps is to slow down. Fast-paced living keeps the brain and nervous system in a state of heightened alertness, making it difficult to tune into internal experiences. Practices that anchor your attention— like mindful breathing, body scans, or gentle movement—help quiet the external noise. These moments of stillness create space for the body's subtle language to emerge.

Mindfulness doesn't require hours of meditation; it can be as simple as noticing your posture while sitting, observing the rhythm of your breath, or tuning in to the taste and texture of your food. This presence builds awareness of habitual patterns—where tension resides, how energy fluctuates, which foods or activities support or drain you. This self-knowledge is empowering because it transforms vague discomfort into actionable insight.

Reconnection also means honoring your body's rhythms. Many people operate on schedules imposed by work, family, or technology rather than their own natural cycles. Paying attention to when you feel most alert, when hunger arises, and when fatigue signals a need for rest invites alignment with your internal clock. This alignment enhances energy, mood, and overall well-being.

Physical sensations themselves are rich sources of information. Pain, for example, is often seen only as a problem to fix, but it can also indicate where healing is needed or where boundaries have been crossed. Learning to differentiate types of pain—sharp, dull, aching, burning— along with the context in which it arises, helps you respond wisely rather than react impulsively.

Hunger and fullness cues are another vital language. Diet culture and emotional eating often sever the connection to these signals, leading to overeating, undereating, or eating for reasons unrelated to true hunger. Restoring trust in your body's ability to guide food intake promotes better digestion, nutrient absorption, and metabolic balance.

Emotional states also manifest physically, and reconnecting means acknowledging how feelings show up in your body. Stress may create tightness in the shoulders, a fluttering heart, or digestive upset. Joy can bring lightness and ease. Recognizing these connections deepens self-understanding and opens pathways to holistic healing.

Technology can be both a help and a hindrance in this process. Wearable devices and apps offer data on sleep, heart rate, and activity, providing objective feedback that complements subjective awareness. However, excessive reliance on data without tuning into internal sensations can perpetuate disconnection. The key is balance—using tools to enhance, not replace, embodied wisdom.

Reconnecting also requires creating safe environments that support listening. Chronic stress, toxic relationships, or environments filled with noise and distraction make it hard to tune in. Setting boundaries around work, social media, and interpersonal interactions protects your capacity for presence and self-care.

Ultimately, this reconnection is a practice of self-compassion. Your body's signals are not inconvenient obstacles but messages of care. Responding with kindness rather than criticism builds trust and opens the door to healing. It's a journey of rediscovery—a return home to yourself.

Building this connection takes time and consistent practice, but the rewards are profound. As you become more attuned, you'll notice patterns and insights emerging—times when your energy dips, foods that ignite or soothe inflammation, emotional triggers that manifest physically. These observations are invaluable for guiding choices that support healing rather than perpetuating imbalance.

Physical movement itself is a powerful tool for reconnecting. Practices like yoga, tai chi, or simple stretching invite you to explore sensations with awareness. They cultivate a sense of embodiment that goes beyond intellectual understanding. Movement allows you to feel where tension holds, where breath is shallow, and where vitality flows. It's a direct dialogue with your body's wisdom.

Breath is another gateway. Often overlooked or shallow, conscious breathing shifts the nervous system from fight-or-flight into relaxation, enhancing your capacity to notice subtle signals. Taking even a few moments daily to observe and deepen your breath rewires stress responses and cultivates calm presence.

Reconnecting also invites curiosity about discomfort rather than avoidance. Instead of pushing through pain or ignoring fatigue, learn to inquire: What might this sensation be trying to tell me? Is it a boundary that needs honoring? Is it a sign of imbalance or depletion? This compassionate inquiry transforms your experience and empowers you to act with care.

Technology can support this process when used mindfully. Journaling apps, symptom trackers, or wearable devices offer objective data that, when paired with subjective awareness, create a fuller picture of your health. They help validate feelings and provide clues about triggers or improvements. Yet, balance is key—technology should never replace your inner wisdom.

Social support also plays a role. Sharing your journey with others who value body awareness fosters encouragement and accountability. Group classes focused on mindfulness or movement, support groups, or simply trusted friends provide space to express and reflect, reinforcing connection.

As you deepen your relationship with your body's signals, you may find old beliefs and judgments surface—messages that you're weak for feeling tired, or that pain means failure. Reframing these beliefs with kindness is essential. Your body is not your enemy. It is the truest friend you have, speaking in a language of sensations and feelings.

Learning to respond rather than react to these signals cultivates resilience. For example, recognizing early fatigue and choosing rest prevents deeper crashes. Noticing digestive discomfort and adjusting your diet avoids inflammation flare-ups. These proactive responses shift you from a reactive cycle of symptoms to a proactive rhythm of self-care.

This reconnection is not about perfection or constant vigilance. It's about presence, patience, and trust. There will be times when you misread signals or ignore them, and that's okay. Healing is a journey, not a destination.

Ultimately, tuning into your body's wisdom fosters empowerment. You no longer feel at the mercy of mysterious symptoms or confusing advice. Instead, you become an active participant in your healing, equipped with the knowledge and compassion to make choices that honor your unique needs.

Reconnecting to your body's signals is reclaiming your voice within— one that guides you toward balance, vitality, and peace. It's an invitation to live fully embodied, aligned with your true self, and free from the noise of disconnection.

# Part III — Your Reset Protocols

After understanding the hidden causes of chronic symptoms and breaking free from the cycles of inflammation, fatigue, and hormonal imbalance, it's time to take intentional action. Part III is where theory meets practice, where knowledge transforms into clear, manageable steps tailored to your unique healing journey.

These reset protocols are designed not as rigid rules but as adaptable frameworks—blueprints you can personalize according to your needs, lifestyle, and progress. They focus on nurturing your body's innate ability to restore balance by addressing foundational pillars: nutrition, movement, sleep, stress management, and mindful reconnection.

Resetting your health is not about perfection or quick fixes. It's about consistency, compassion, and respect for the complex interplay within your body. Each protocol aims to empower you to rebuild resilience steadily and sustainably, avoiding overwhelm and burnout.

In this part, you will find actionable guidance to help recalibrate your system—whether that means rebuilding gut health, stabilizing blood sugar, restoring hormonal harmony, or cultivating restful sleep. The goal is to create a supportive environment where your body can heal deeply and naturally.

Embrace this chapter as an invitation to reclaim agency over your health, to move beyond frustration, and to cultivate lasting vitality. The journey ahead is one of discovery, renewal, and empowerment—your reset protocols are the tools to guide you home.

# Chapter 10: The Mind-Body Repair Process

## Your Nervous System and Trauma Response

The nervous system is the silent conductor of your body's orchestra, governing everything from heartbeat to digestion, sleep to immune function. It constantly monitors the environment for signs of safety or threat, adjusting your body's responses accordingly. While this system is designed to protect you, modern life and unresolved emotional experiences can push it into a persistent state of hypervigilance—where the trauma response becomes stuck, affecting your health in profound ways.

Trauma doesn't only refer to dramatic or obvious events. It can be the accumulation of everyday stressors, emotional wounds, neglect, or experiences that overwhelm your capacity to cope. When trauma occurs, your nervous system activates survival mechanisms: fight, flight, freeze, or collapse. These responses trigger a cascade of physiological changes—elevated heart rate, rapid breathing, cortisol release—that prepare you to face immediate danger.

The problem arises when this survival mode lingers long after the danger has passed. The nervous system remains locked in a state of alert, perceiving threats in benign situations. This chronic activation disrupts the delicate balance between the sympathetic nervous system (responsible for fight or flight) and the parasympathetic system (responsible for rest and repair). When the sympathetic tone dominates, your body stays in a heightened state of stress, which fuels inflammation, disrupts hormone balance, impairs digestion, and fragments sleep.

Understanding this is crucial because many chronic health issues—fatigue, brain fog, digestive problems, autoimmune flare-ups—are linked to this persistent trauma response. Your body is not malfunctioning randomly; it is responding logically to perceived threats. The nervous system's overactivation is often the root cause keeping symptoms alive.

Healing the nervous system and trauma response means creating space for your body to shift from survival to safety. This shift isn't about simply "relaxing" or "thinking positive." It requires intentional practices that regulate your nervous system at a deep level and gently retrain it to recognize safety again.

One foundational approach involves **mindful awareness**—learning to observe sensations, emotions, and thoughts without judgment. This cultivates a sense of presence that helps break cycles of fear and avoidance. It teaches your nervous system that you can tolerate discomfort and uncertainty without reacting with alarm.

Breathwork is another powerful tool. Since breath is both voluntary and involuntary, it serves as a bridge between conscious control and autonomic regulation. Slow, deep, rhythmic breathing activates the parasympathetic nervous system, lowering heart rate and cortisol levels, and promoting a state conducive to healing.

Movement practices like yoga, tai chi, or gentle stretching also support nervous system regulation. They engage proprioception—the body's sense of position and movement—which grounds you in the present and calms hyperarousal. Movement becomes not only physical exercise but a form of embodied mindfulness.

Somatic therapies, which focus on body awareness and releasing stored tension, can unlock trauma held deep within muscles and connective tissue. These approaches recognize that trauma is often "trapped" physically, and healing requires more than talk—it requires sensing and moving through held patterns.

Creating safe environments—both external and internal—is essential. This means setting boundaries in relationships, reducing sensory overload, and cultivating self-compassion. The nervous system needs repeated experiences of safety to rewire and reset.

It's important to remember that healing from trauma is rarely linear. Progress often unfolds in waves, with periods of discomfort as buried emotions surface. This is a natural part of the process, signaling that your nervous system is learning new patterns.

The journey toward healing your nervous system also involves learning how to recognize and honor your body's limits. Many people live in a state of pushing past exhaustion, ignoring subtle signs that their nervous system is overwhelmed. This chronic overdrive keeps the trauma response active and prevents restoration. Embracing rest—not as laziness but as an essential act of self-care—allows your system the time it needs to downshift from survival mode.

Practices that foster **co-regulation**—sharing calm and safety through connection—are invaluable. Whether through trusted relationships, therapy, or supportive community, feeling seen and safe with others sends powerful signals to your nervous system. This social safety promotes healing in ways solo efforts cannot replicate.

Mind-body approaches that integrate breath, movement, and mindfulness, such as somatic experiencing, EMDR (Eye Movement Desensitization and Reprocessing), or trauma-informed yoga, offer pathways to process trauma without retraumatization. These modalities work gently with your body's natural rhythms, helping release stored tension and rebuild nervous system flexibility.

It's also important to acknowledge that trauma lives not just in the nervous system but also in your beliefs and narratives. Often, trauma imprints limiting stories—"I'm not safe," "I'm not enough," or "I must always be strong." These narratives reinforce hypervigilance and stress responses. Healing involves reshaping these internal scripts with compassion and evidence of safety, a process often supported by therapy or guided self-inquiry.

The physical symptoms of trauma response—tight muscles, digestive issues, insomnia, immune dysregulation—are signals, not diagnoses. Recognizing them as such shifts your perspective from frustration or fear toward curiosity and empowerment. You become an active participant in decoding and responding to your body's messages.

Healing your nervous system is not a quick fix. It unfolds over weeks, months, or even years, depending on the depth and duration of trauma. Patience is essential. Progress may be slow or nonlinear, but each step toward safety and regulation compounds over time, building resilience and restoring balance.

Integrating these approaches creates a foundation not just for symptom relief but for a profound transformation. As your nervous system learns to trust safety again, inflammation reduces, hormonal rhythms stabilize, sleep improves, and energy returns. Mental clarity and emotional resilience deepen. You reclaim your body as a safe and trustworthy ally.

Ultimately, addressing trauma and nervous system dysregulation is one of the most powerful acts of self-healing. It honors the intimate connection between mind and body, recognizing that true wellness requires harmony between the two. By embracing this journey with compassion and intention, you open the door to lasting health, balance, and vitality.

# Chronic Stress and the Mind-Body Loop

Stress is an unavoidable part of life, a natural response to challenges that prepare us to act and adapt. In small doses, stress is healthy—it sharpens focus, boosts energy, and motivates problem-solving. However, when stress becomes chronic, lingering without resolution, it transforms into a silent saboteur, disrupting every system in the body and mind. Understanding the intricate mind-body loop of chronic stress is essential for breaking free from its grip and restoring health.

The mind and body are not separate entities but deeply intertwined. Thoughts, emotions, and perceptions influence physical responses, while bodily sensations feedback to shape mental states. Chronic stress activates this loop continuously, keeping the nervous system in a state of heightened alert. This persistent activation floods the body with stress hormones like cortisol and adrenaline, which, over time, wear down resilience.

Cortisol, while vital for short-term survival, becomes damaging when elevated chronically. It impairs immune function, increases inflammation, disrupts blood sugar regulation, and interferes with sleep. The brain regions responsible for memory, emotional regulation, and decision-making shrink under prolonged cortisol exposure, while the amygdala—the fear center—becomes hyperactive. This neurochemical imbalance fuels anxiety, depression, and cognitive fog.

Physically, chronic stress manifests in diverse symptoms: muscle tension, digestive disturbances, headaches, fatigue, and hormonal disruptions. Because the mind-body loop perpetuates itself, these physical symptoms often reinforce mental stress, creating a feedback cycle that feels impossible to escape. The more your body reacts, the more your mind worries, which triggers more physical distress.

One key element in this loop is the perception of threat. The brain does not distinguish well between physical danger and psychological stressors like work pressure, relationship conflicts, or financial worries. Both activate the same survival pathways, triggering fight, flight, or freeze responses. For those experiencing chronic stress, the brain essentially remains stuck in "emergency mode," unable to shift into rest and repair. The autonomic nervous system, which regulates involuntary functions like heart rate and digestion, is central to this dynamic. It consists of the sympathetic nervous system—responsible for the stress response—and the parasympathetic nervous system, which promotes relaxation and healing. Chronic stress skews this balance, favoring sympathetic dominance and suppressing parasympathetic activity. This imbalance disrupts digestion, immune regulation, and sleep, undermining the body's ability to recover.

Breaking the chronic stress cycle requires both mental and physical strategies that address this mind-body interaction. Awareness is the first step—recognizing when stress is affecting not only your mood but also your physical well-being. Often, people compartmentalize emotions and bodily symptoms, missing the connection that could guide effective healing.

Mindfulness practices help cultivate this awareness. By observing thoughts and sensations without judgment, you create space to respond rather than react. This gentle witnessing reduces the intensity of stress reactions and retrains the nervous system toward balance. Breathwork, which directly influences the autonomic nervous system, offers another powerful tool to calm the mind-body loop.

Lifestyle factors profoundly influence your capacity to manage chronic stress. Sleep, nutrition, movement, and social connection either buffer or exacerbate the stress response. For example, poor sleep increases cortisol production, fueling the cycle, while regular movement supports parasympathetic activation and emotional resilience.

Mental habits also shape the loop. Negative thought patterns, perfectionism, and unresolved emotional conflicts amplify stress signals. Cultivating self-compassion and cognitive flexibility can weaken these patterns, creating more adaptive responses to life's challenges.

Interrupting this cycle means creating consistent, supportive habits that recalibrate both mind and body. It's not about eliminating stress altogether—that's impossible—but about increasing your capacity to manage and recover from stress in healthier ways. Small, intentional practices can shift the nervous system from constant fight-or-flight to a state of rest and repair.

Regular mindfulness meditation is one of the most effective tools for this transformation. It trains the brain to observe stress triggers without becoming overwhelmed, reducing amygdala hyperactivity and strengthening areas involved in emotional regulation. Even short daily sessions, practiced with patience, produce measurable improvements in stress resilience.

Physical movement plays a complementary role. Gentle, rhythmic activities like walking, swimming, or yoga activate the parasympathetic nervous system and increase endorphin production, lifting mood and calming anxiety. Unlike high-intensity workouts, which can sometimes exacerbate stress if overdone, these forms of movement nurture balance and connection to your body.

Nutrition is equally vital. Chronic stress depletes key nutrients like magnesium, B vitamins, and omega-3 fatty acids, which are necessary for nervous system function and stress modulation. Prioritizing whole, nutrient-dense foods helps replenish these stores, supporting biochemical pathways that promote calm and recovery.

Sleep hygiene cannot be overstated. Deep, restorative sleep resets the mind-body loop, clearing stress hormones and repairing neural pathways. Establishing consistent routines, reducing screen time before bed, and creating a soothing environment are foundational for restoring sleep quality.

Social support and connection are powerful buffers against chronic stress. Human beings are wired for connection, and feeling supported mitigates the perception of threat that drives the stress response. Sharing your experiences with trusted friends, family, or therapists provides emotional validation and helps regulate your nervous system through co-regulation.

Cognitive strategies also matter. Challenging unhelpful thought patterns, practicing gratitude, and cultivating self-compassion reduce mental stress and interrupt the feedback loop that fuels physical symptoms.

Journaling or therapy can facilitate this internal work, providing space to process emotions and develop new perspectives.

Importantly, addressing chronic stress requires recognizing and honoring your limits. Overcommitting or ignoring early warning signs perpetuates burnout. Learning to say no, setting boundaries, and prioritizing rest are acts of courage and self-respect essential for healing. This integrated approach—combining mindfulness, movement, nutrition, sleep, social support, and cognitive work—does more than alleviate symptoms. It rewires your nervous system, restoring flexibility and balance. Over time, your body and mind learn to coexist in harmony, enabling you to respond to life's challenges with resilience rather than exhaustion.

Healing chronic stress is a journey, not a quick fix. Progress may be gradual, with setbacks and breakthroughs. Patience and self-compassion are your allies. Each step toward balance strengthens your mind-body connection and builds the foundation for lasting health.

By understanding the profound impact of chronic stress on your physiology and psyche, and by embracing practices that nurture regulation, you reclaim control over your well-being. You transform stress from an unrelenting burden into a manageable part of life—one that no longer dictates your health or happiness.

# The Power of Awareness in Healing

Healing is often seen as a purely physical process—taking supplements, changing diets, or following treatment plans. But true healing runs far deeper, beginning with awareness. Awareness is the foundation upon which transformation builds. It is the conscious recognition of your body, mind, emotions, and environment—an intentional noticing that opens the door to change.

When you cultivate awareness, you step out of autopilot. Instead of reacting unconsciously to symptoms or stressors, you observe your experiences with curiosity and clarity. This shift—from being overwhelmed by what's happening to simply witnessing it—creates space for insight and choice. Suddenly, patterns that once seemed automatic or mysterious become understandable and manageable.

Awareness is not about judgment or criticism. It is a gentle, compassionate attention that accepts where you are without demanding immediate fixes. This acceptance is crucial because resistance often fuels stress and tension, blocking progress. When you acknowledge your current reality with kindness, you reduce internal conflict and invite healing energy to flow.

Your body sends countless signals every moment—tightness in muscles, fluctuations in energy, digestive sensations, emotional shifts. These signals are your personal language, conveying what your system needs or warning you of imbalance. Learning to tune into these messages deepens your connection to self and guides you toward choices that support restoration rather than further depletion.

Mindfulness practices are one of the most effective ways to develop this awareness. Simple exercises—like focusing on your breath, observing sensations without reaction, or tuning into your emotions—train your brain to be present. This presence reduces anxiety and rewires neural pathways associated with stress, fostering calm and clarity.

Beyond formal mindfulness, everyday moments offer opportunities to practice awareness. Noticing how your body feels during meals, observing how certain environments impact your mood, or reflecting on the quality of your sleep can all provide valuable data. This ongoing feedback loop helps you tailor your lifestyle to your unique needs rather than following generic advice.

Awareness also shines light on the emotional and mental layers of healing. Often, unresolved feelings or limiting beliefs maintain chronic symptoms. By becoming aware of these hidden factors—without pushing them away or becoming consumed—you empower yourself to work through them. Emotional awareness can be a catalyst for releasing stuck energy and restoring balance.

This process requires patience. Early on, awareness may reveal discomfort or uncertainty. You might uncover habits or patterns that are difficult to face. Yet, this is the paradox of healing: the very act of noticing discomfort begins to soften its hold. Over time, what once felt overwhelming becomes manageable.

Importantly, awareness expands beyond internal experiences to include your relationship with the world. How do your daily routines, relationships, and environments support or stress you? By observing these external factors, you gain insight into adjustments that can reduce strain and enhance well-being.

True healing is holistic. Awareness integrates body, mind, and environment into a cohesive understanding. It transforms passive suffering into active engagement, turning symptoms from obstacles into guides.

As awareness deepens, it fosters a profound sense of empowerment. No longer a passive recipient of symptoms or external circumstances, you become an active participant in your healing journey. This shift from victimhood to agency changes everything. With each observation, you gain clarity about what nourishes you and what depletes you, enabling more informed choices that align with your body's true needs.

Awareness also cultivates resilience. When you understand your triggers—whether physical, emotional, or environmental—you can prepare and respond rather than be blindsided. This preparedness reduces the intensity and duration of flare-ups, lessening their impact on your life. Over time, this proactive relationship with your health fosters confidence and reduces anxiety about symptoms.

Importantly, this power comes with compassion. Awareness is not about self-criticism or striving for perfection. It's a gentle presence that recognizes healing is non-linear, often messy, and deeply personal. There will be days of clarity and days of confusion. Moments of progress may be followed by setbacks. Maintaining a compassionate stance allows you to navigate this ebb and flow without judgment, keeping you engaged and motivated.

In practical terms, cultivating awareness can be supported through tools like journaling, where writing about your experiences illuminates patterns and emotional currents. Tracking symptoms alongside lifestyle factors reveals connections you might otherwise miss. This documentation becomes a dialogue between you and your body, an ongoing conversation that guides your path.

Another way awareness aids healing is by breaking automatic cycles. Many patterns—overeating, negative self-talk, sedentary habits—occur unconsciously. Bringing these into conscious view interrupts their momentum, creating opportunities for change. This mindful interruption is a powerful form of self-care.

Connection to your body's signals also enhances intuition. As you become fluent in your internal language, you learn to trust your instincts about what feels right or wrong, safe or risky. This inner guidance can steer you away from quick fixes or harmful habits, directing you toward choices that support sustainable well-being.

Furthermore, awareness fosters a sense of gratitude and appreciation for your body's resilience. Even in the midst of illness or discomfort, noticing moments of ease, strength, or healing reinforces hope and nurtures a positive mindset. This positivity is itself a healing force, influencing neurochemical balance and immune function.

The power of awareness extends into relationships as well. Being present with others—listening deeply, communicating authentically—creates emotional safety and support that buffer stress. These social connections are vital for health and healing, reminding you that you are not alone.

Ultimately, awareness is the gateway to integration—bringing mind, body, and environment into harmony. It dissolves the false boundaries that separate physical symptoms from emotional experience, empowering you to approach healing holistically. Through awareness, what once felt like chaos begins to reveal its hidden order, guiding you toward balance and vitality.

Embracing awareness means embracing yourself fully—with all your complexities, vulnerabilities, and strengths. It invites you to meet your healing journey with openness and kindness, transforming every sensation, thought, and feeling into a teacher. This is the foundation for lasting change and a vibrant life well lived.

# Part IV — Redefining Health

As you move deeper into your healing journey, you begin to realize that health is far more than the absence of symptoms. It is a dynamic, evolving state—one that encompasses physical vitality, emotional balance, mental clarity, and a meaningful connection to yourself and the world around you. This final part invites you to expand your understanding and redefine what health truly means for you.

Redefining health challenges conventional narratives that focus solely on fixing problems or eradicating disease. Instead, it encourages a holistic, integrative approach that honors the complexity and uniqueness of your body and life experience. It embraces wellness as a process of continual growth, self-awareness, and alignment with your authentic needs and values.

In this section, you will explore principles and practices that support not only healing but thriving. You will discover how to cultivate resilience in the face of life's inevitable challenges and develop sustainable habits that nurture your well-being across all dimensions—physical, emotional, and spiritual.

This is your invitation to step into a new relationship with health—one that is empowering, compassionate, and grounded in real-world practicality. As you redefine health on your own terms, you reclaim the power to live fully, vibrantly, and authentically.

# Chapter 11: Reclaiming Wholeness

## Why You're Not Broken

In the journey through chronic symptoms, fatigue, or mental fog, it's easy to feel as if your body has betrayed you—that something inside is fundamentally broken or defective. This belief can create a heavy burden, adding shame, frustration, and hopelessness to the physical and emotional challenges you face. But the truth is profoundly different: you are not broken. Your body is responding with remarkable intelligence to the circumstances it has encountered, and healing is not about fixing a broken machine—it's about restoring balance to a dynamic system.

The human body is a resilient, adaptive organism designed to handle stress, recover from injury, and maintain equilibrium. When symptoms arise, they are signals—messages indicating that the body's current environment or inputs are out of alignment with its needs. Rather than evidence of failure, symptoms are evidence of the body's ongoing effort to protect and heal itself.

Consider inflammation, often seen as a villain. In reality, it is a critical defense mechanism—a complex biological response to injury or threat. Chronic inflammation is not a sign that your body is broken but that it is stuck in a prolonged state of vigilance, often due to unresolved stressors, environmental toxins, or lifestyle factors. Recognizing this reframes your experience from one of defectiveness to one of survival and adaptation.

Similarly, fatigue is often misunderstood as weakness. Fatigue is the body's way of signaling that energy resources are depleted or diverted to healing processes. It's a protective measure urging rest and restoration. Viewing fatigue through this lens invites compassion for yourself rather than self-judgment.

The notion that you're broken can also stem from the medical model's focus on disease and pathology. When health care emphasizes symptoms as problems to be eradicated without exploring root causes, it can inadvertently reinforce feelings of brokenness. This is why a shift toward a holistic, systems-based understanding is so important—it sees you as a whole person, not a collection of faulty parts.

Your body's responses are shaped by a lifetime of experiences— genetics, environment, diet, stress, trauma, and choices. Healing is the process of gently addressing these layers, removing obstacles, and providing support. It's less about "fixing" and more about rebalancing.

This perspective empowers you. It acknowledges your body's wisdom and invites you to become an active collaborator in your healing. Instead of passively enduring symptoms or chasing quick fixes, you learn to listen, interpret, and respond to your body's signals with care and respect.

There is no universal standard for "perfect" health. Each person's baseline and journey are unique. What looks like limitation or dysfunction from one angle is often an adaptive response from another. Embracing this complexity frees you from unrealistic expectations and harsh self-criticism.

Healing is not about erasing your history or forcing your body into an idealized version of health. It's about honoring where you've been, recognizing the adaptations your body has made to protect you, and partnering with it to create new patterns of balance and vitality. This shift in perspective opens the door to self-compassion—a vital ingredient in any healing journey.

Self-compassion allows you to see your symptoms not as personal failings but as understandable responses to life's challenges. It encourages patience with setbacks and perseverance through frustration. When you stop fighting against your body and begin listening to it with kindness, you create a nurturing environment where change can flourish.

It's also important to remember that healing is rarely linear or quick. Your body is rewiring, recalibrating, and rebuilding systems that may have been under stress for months or years. This process requires time, consistent care, and sometimes trial and error. Recognizing this helps temper expectations and reduce the pressure to achieve immediate results.

Alongside patience, curiosity becomes a powerful ally. Asking questions like "What is my body trying to tell me?" or "Which parts of my lifestyle support or hinder my healing?" transforms your role from passive sufferer to active investigator. This curiosity uncovers hidden connections and empowers you to make informed decisions that align with your unique biology.

Modern health paradigms often overlook this individualized, adaptive nature of the body. They tend to promote one-size-fits-all solutions that can leave you feeling blamed or inadequate when results don't match promises. Redefining your health narrative to one of resilience rather than brokenness liberates you from these external pressures.

Your body's complexity means it communicates in layers—physical symptoms, emotional signals, and energetic shifts. Healing requires tuning into this rich language, integrating all dimensions rather than isolating parts. When you embrace this wholeness, you move toward health that is vibrant, sustainable, and deeply rooted in your own experience.

It's also helpful to acknowledge the strength it takes to endure chronic symptoms and still seek solutions. Your persistence and willingness to engage in your healing journey demonstrate resilience and courage. This strength is the foundation on which lasting transformation is built.

Ultimately, you are not broken—you are whole, dynamic, and capable of profound healing. Your symptoms are not signs of failure but invitations to listen more deeply and respond with greater wisdom. Embracing this truth frees you to move beyond despair and into a space of hope, agency, and renewal.

This mindset shifts the focus from fixing deficits to nurturing growth. It honors the complexity of human health and the interplay of body, mind, and environment. It creates room for grace when progress is slow and celebrates every step forward, no matter how small.

In reclaiming your health, remember that you are not alone. Many have walked this path, transforming their understanding of what it means to be well. You too can rewrite your story—not as someone broken, but as someone whole, learning, and evolving.

# How to Become the Expert of Your Own Body

Taking charge of your health starts with becoming deeply familiar with your own body—its rhythms, signals, strengths, and vulnerabilities. While healthcare professionals provide essential guidance and expertise, no one knows your experience better than you do. Becoming the expert of your own body means cultivating an intimate understanding of how it responds to different foods, environments, emotions, and activities, empowering you to make informed choices that foster true healing.

This process begins with intentional observation. Rather than brushing off symptoms or dismissing feelings as insignificant, you start paying attention to patterns—how energy fluctuates throughout the day, which foods trigger discomfort, or how stress affects your digestion. These observations are the raw data of self-knowledge, invaluable for tailoring your lifestyle to your unique needs.

Journaling is a practical tool that supports this exploration. Writing down what you eat, how you sleep, your mood changes, physical sensations, and daily activities creates a map of your health landscape. Over time, connections emerge that might have been hidden beneath the noise of daily life. This record becomes a conversation between you and your body, allowing you to experiment thoughtfully and track progress.

Becoming an expert also involves asking questions—curious, open-ended inquiries rather than rigid demands. What time of day do you feel most energized? Which environments soothe or stress you? How does your body respond after certain meals or movement practices? These questions shift you from passive recipient of advice to active investigator, fostering a sense of agency and empowerment.

Listening to your body's signals requires patience and gentle curiosity. Early on, you might notice discomfort or confusion when tuning into subtle sensations. You may realize that some long-held habits don't serve you well, or that emotional patterns influence physical symptoms. This awareness, though sometimes challenging, is essential for growth.

Understanding your body also means recognizing that it's a dynamic system, not a static machine. What works at one point may need adjustment later. Seasons, life stages, stress levels, and environmental changes all influence your needs. Maintaining an ongoing dialogue with your body ensures that your strategies remain aligned with your current reality.

Education is another pillar of expertise. Learning basic principles of nutrition, physiology, and stress response helps decode the messages your body sends. However, it's important to balance this knowledge with humility—every body is unique, and what applies broadly may not apply specifically to you. Combining education with self-observation creates a powerful synergy.

Developing this expertise takes time, and it's natural to feel overwhelmed by conflicting information. The key is to focus on what resonates with your experience and to experiment slowly, observing results without rushing or forcing outcomes. This measured approach reduces frustration and builds confidence.

Seeking professional support can enhance your journey. Practitioners who respect your lived experience and guide rather than dictate empower you to deepen your understanding. Together, you can interpret symptoms, design personalized strategies, and navigate complexities that arise.

As you deepen your expertise, you develop a finely tuned sense of what supports or challenges your well-being. This knowledge empowers you to advocate for yourself confidently in medical or therapeutic settings. When you understand your patterns and responses, you can ask informed questions, request specific tests, and discern which interventions align with your needs. This collaboration transforms healthcare from a one-sided experience into a partnership.

Being the expert of your own body also means embracing flexibility. Healing is rarely a straight path, and setbacks are natural. Your body may react differently from day to day or as you introduce new practices. Rather than seeing these shifts as failures, view them as signals to adjust and learn. This adaptive mindset prevents discouragement and keeps you engaged in your journey.

Another important aspect is trusting your intuition. Beyond observable symptoms and scientific knowledge lies a deeper internal knowing. As you cultivate awareness and understanding, you become more attuned to subtle cues—what feels nourishing or draining, when to push forward or rest. Honoring this intuitive wisdom balances external information with personal experience, creating a holistic approach.

Developing expertise also involves recognizing your limits and when to seek outside help. Self-knowledge does not mean going it alone. Sometimes, professional guidance is essential to navigate complex health issues or emotional challenges. The key is to choose practitioners who honor your experience, listen deeply, and support your autonomy.

Technology and tools can assist in this process. Wearables, symptom trackers, or apps provide objective data that complement subjective awareness. These tools can reveal trends or triggers you might miss and support more precise adjustments. However, it's important not to become overly reliant on devices—your internal experience remains the primary guide.

Over time, becoming your own expert shifts your relationship with health from reactive to proactive. You move beyond simply managing symptoms to cultivating conditions that foster thriving. This perspective inspires you to prioritize prevention, self-care, and ongoing learning.

The journey of self-expertise is also deeply personal and transformative. It reconnects you with your body as a wise, responsive partner rather than a problem to be solved. This reconnection nurtures self-compassion, resilience, and empowerment.

Remember, expertise is not about perfection or having all the answers. It's about cultivating curiosity, openness, and trust in your capacity to understand and care for yourself. Every small insight, every observation, builds a richer, more nuanced map of your health.

Ultimately, you hold the most important knowledge for your healing—your lived experience. By becoming the expert of your own body, you reclaim power, foster deeper healing, and create a foundation for lasting well-being that aligns with your unique life.

# Building a New Definition of Health

Health is often narrowly defined as the absence of disease or the ability to perform certain physical tasks. This traditional view, while useful in acute medical contexts, falls short in capturing the full spectrum of human well-being. For many living with chronic symptoms or complex health challenges, health feels elusive or out of reach. Building a new definition of health is essential—a perspective that honors the complexity of your experience and embraces wellness as a dynamic, evolving state.

This new definition begins by recognizing health as more than physical metrics. It integrates emotional balance, mental clarity, social connection, and a sense of purpose. Health becomes a holistic interplay of body, mind, and environment—a continuous process rather than a fixed destination.

One cornerstone of this redefinition is embracing health as resilience. Resilience is the capacity to adapt and recover from stress, setbacks, and change. It acknowledges that life includes challenges, but your ability to navigate them with grace and strength is a measure of wellness. This reframing shifts the focus from eliminating all symptoms to cultivating balance and flexibility.

Another key element is personalization. Health is not one-size-fits-all. What nourishes one person might not suit another. Genetics, life history, environment, and values all shape your unique health blueprint. Building a new definition means honoring this individuality, moving away from rigid norms toward a more fluid understanding.

This perspective also invites you to value progress over perfection. Wellness is rarely linear, especially when recovering from chronic issues. Fluctuations, plateaus, and occasional setbacks are natural parts of the journey. Recognizing these patterns as normal helps reduce frustration and sustain motivation.

The new definition encourages a deep connection with your body's wisdom. Instead of viewing symptoms solely as problems to fix, it sees them as messages guiding you toward balance. This relationship fosters curiosity and compassion, transforming healing into an act of partnership with yourself.

Social and environmental factors also belong in this expanded view. Supportive relationships, meaningful work, safe living spaces, and connection to nature all profoundly impact health. Acknowledging these influences broadens your toolkit beyond diet and exercise to include lifestyle and community.

Importantly, this redefinition values mental and emotional health as foundational, not secondary. Anxiety, depression, or unresolved trauma affect physical well-being profoundly. Prioritizing mental health practices—such as mindfulness, therapy, or creative expression—strengthens overall resilience and vitality.

As you build this new definition, you also reclaim agency. Instead of feeling at the mercy of symptoms or external judgments, you become an active participant in shaping your well-being. This empowerment fuels hope and commitment.

Embracing this broader definition invites a shift from viewing health as a static goal to seeing it as a lifelong journey. It's a path of continual learning, adaptation, and self-discovery. Your body and mind will evolve with time, and so will your understanding of what wellness means for you at each stage of life.

This approach also encourages you to honor small victories and everyday moments of well-being. Perhaps it's waking up with more ease, enjoying a walk without discomfort, or finding moments of peace amid chaos. These glimpses of balance are meaningful milestones, reminding you that health is not an all-or-nothing state but a spectrum of experience.

Building a new definition also challenges societal pressures that equate health with productivity or appearance. True wellness respects your intrinsic worth beyond external achievements or aesthetics. It prioritizes self-care, rest, and joy as legitimate and essential components of a healthy life.

Mindfulness and presence become vital tools in this process. By tuning into your current state without judgment, you cultivate a compassionate relationship with yourself. This awareness helps you recognize when to push forward and when to pause, creating a sustainable rhythm that honors your needs.

Community and connection also play a crucial role. Sharing your journey with others who understand and support your vision of health provides encouragement and reduces isolation. Collective wisdom often enriches personal insight, creating a supportive environment for transformation.

This redefinition encourages curiosity about what health can be, inviting experimentation and flexibility. Rather than rigid adherence to strict rules, it promotes listening to your body and adapting practices as needed. This responsiveness nurtures resilience and reduces the risk of burnout.

Finally, building this new health paradigm empowers you to rewrite your story. You move from seeing yourself as a passive victim of illness to an active co-creator of wellness. This narrative shift ignites hope, motivation, and a deep sense of agency that sustains your healing over time.

In embracing a new definition of health, you reclaim your power to live authentically and vibrantly. You honor the complexity of your being and the richness of your experience, creating a foundation for lasting well-being that is uniquely yours.